yoga
pilates

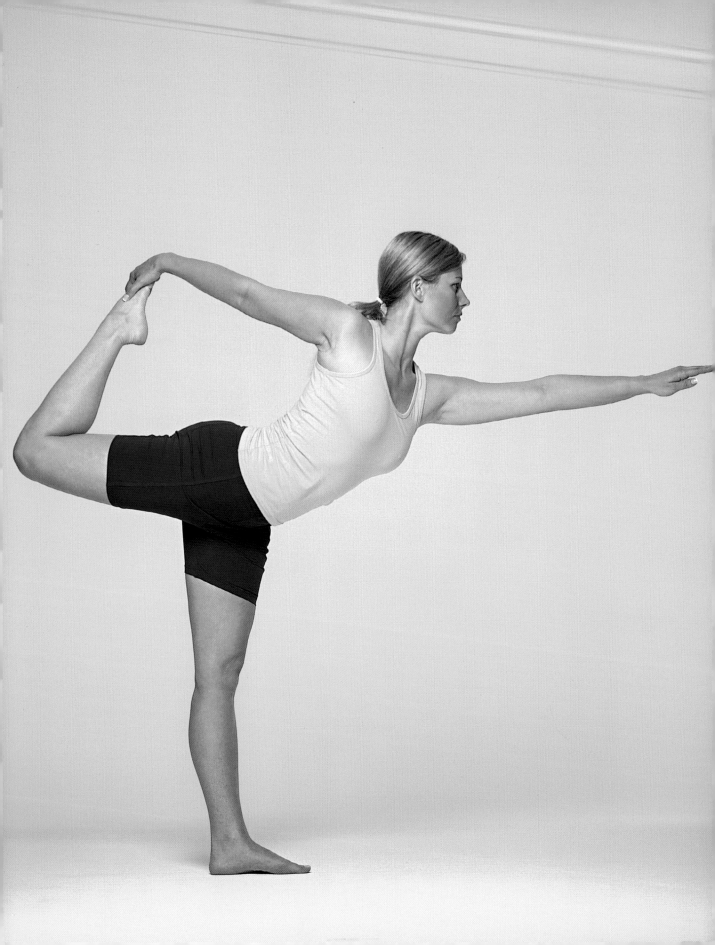

yoga pilates

a balanced workout for healthy living

Jacqueline Lysycia

GRAMERCY BOOKS NEW YORK

Copyright © 2005 Octopus Publishing Group

This 2005 edition is published by Gramercy Books, an imprint of Random House Value Publishing, a division of Random House, Inc., New York, by arrangement with Mitchell Beazley, Octopus Publishing Group, London.

Gramercy is a registered trademark and the colophon is a trademark of Random House, Inc.

Random House
New York • Toronto • London • Sydney • Auckland
www.randomhouse.com

Printed and bound in China

A catalog record for this title is available from the Library of Congress.

ISBN 0-517-22442-9

10 9 8 7 6 5 4 3 2 1

Contents

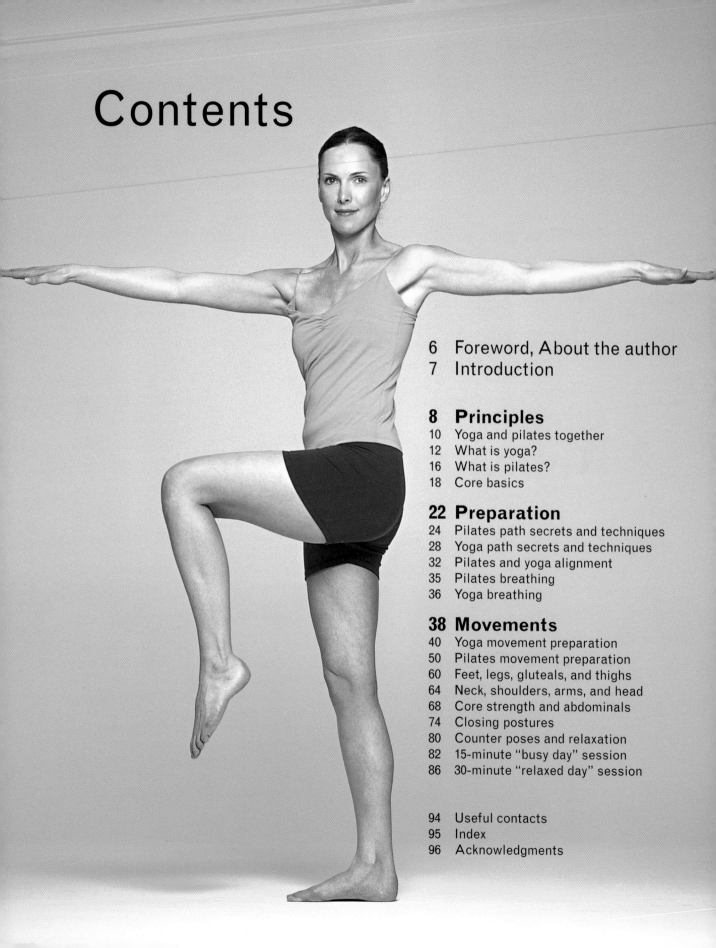

foreword

This book has taken me over five years to compile, and my travels to uncover the sympathetic practice of yoga and pilates have taken me all the way around the world. Inspired by the thousands of students that I teach globally, I wanted to find a way of illustrating the clear similarities and differences that exist between yoga and pilates and how they can be used for maximum health and well-being.

Although yoga and pilates originate from vastly different cultures and philosophies, they do share many of the same benefits and characteristics. Both disciplines can work alongside each other very effectively, as long as the clear distinctions are understood. Pilates can add much value to yoga practice, and vice versa, without the integrity of either practice being lost. The method I have developed opens up an exciting way of exercising without diluting either form.

Thank you to all my students for their discipline and loyalty, and especially to my teachers for sharing their wisdom, understanding, and experience so I could produce a book that I wish I had read years ago. Enjoy!

about the author

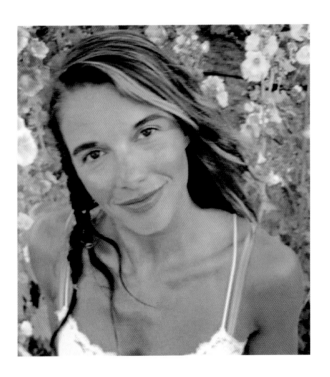

Jacqueline Lysycia is a certified yoga and pilates teacher and a Master Reebok Trainer with her own studio space in Essex where she practices and teaches. She is Co-Director of Yoga in Schools UK and oversees the training and accreditation for pilates teachers across Europe.

Jacqueline has studied with many masters of Dynamic, Ashtanga, Iyengar, and Hatha Yoga. Her trademark style is an energizing practice to suit all levels that draws upon the effortless flow of vinyasa, the anatomical alignment of Iyengar, via the dynamic and safe delivery of vinyasa krama.

Jacqueline is the author of *The Pilates Workpack*, *5-Minute Pilates*, and *The 10-Minute Wake-Up Workout* and has worked on several yoga and pilates videos. She is in the process of setting up a yoga school on the beautiful Brac Island in Croatia.

introduction

movement preparation

Before you start your pilates and yoga programme, it is advisable to do the alignment and breathing exercises (see pp.32–7) so that you learn the correct techniques for standing and sitting and engaging the correct muscles according to the instructions given.

Once you have worked through the alignment and breathing exercises you can start with a yoga- or pilates-style warm-up (see pp.40–59). Allow yourself 5–10 minutes to learn each technique and check the instructions before you attempt to warm up as a flowing sequence. It will take a little time to familiarize yourself with the techniques, but it is always best to learn them correctly. If you learn and perform the movements incorrectly you may increase tension, and this can lead to injury.

movements

The movements are split into six sections:
* Feet, legs, gluteals, and thighs
* Neck, shoulders, arms, and head
* Core strength and abdominals
* Closing postures
* Counter poses and relaxation
* 15-minute "busy day" session and 30-minute "relaxed day" session

Each section contains a mixture of yoga and pilates movements offering various levels of difficulty. We advise picking at least two movements or postures from each section depending upon the time you have available. Once you have decided on which movements to practise, learn and perform them according to the instructions. You will find that some movements will take longer to refine than others. Always master the simplest level before moving upwards.

Yoga movements are colour coded blue and pilates movements are colour coded green. Moves that are practiced in both pilates and yoga are identified with this symbol: If you are feeling lethargic just practise the breathing drills (see pp.36–7) and then go into Relaxation Pose (see p.81). Even this short sequence is better than doing nothing at all.

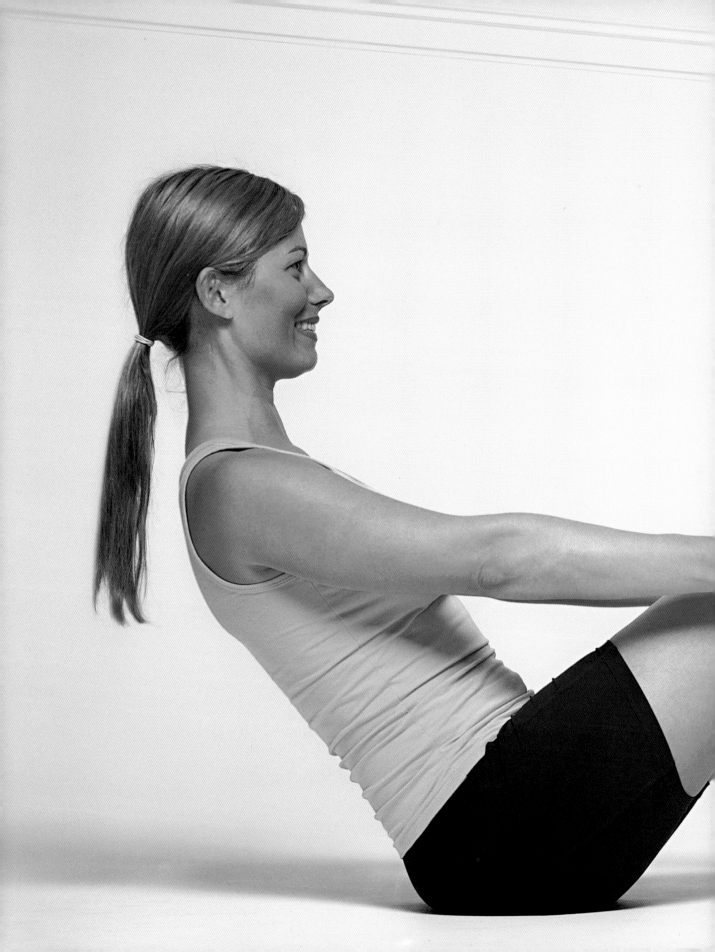

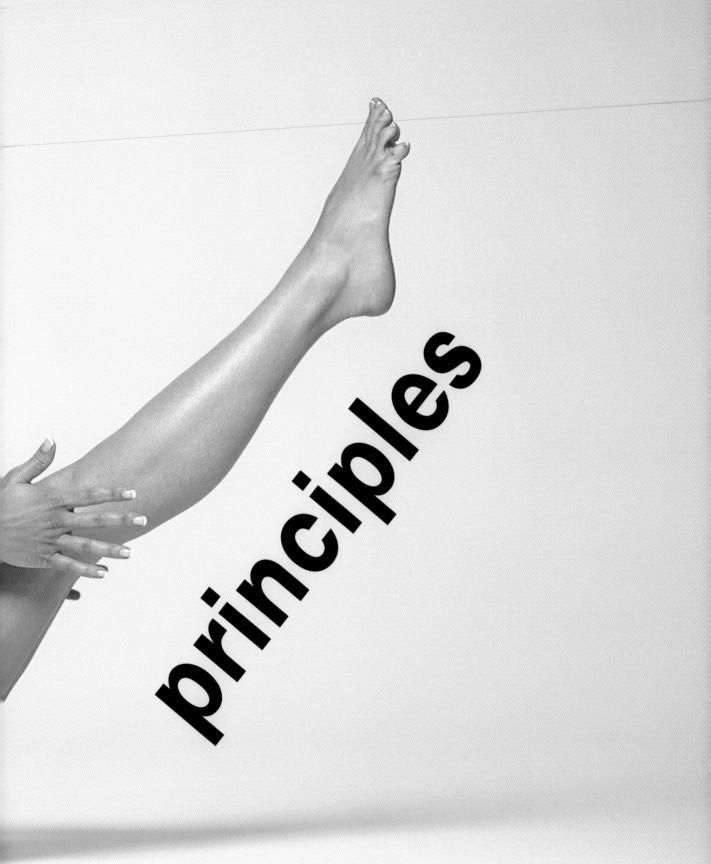

principles

yoga and pilates together

Yogapilates is a very modern approach to movement using the ancient wisdom of yoga and the immune-boosting benefits of pilates. In combination, they provide a fresh approach to living a healthy, active lifestyle in today's pressurized urban world.

Modern life presents us with very different stresses to the times when yoga and pilates were first conceived. *Yogapilates* will teach you to understand the clear associations and distinctions between these two successful forms of movement. It will teach you in layman's terms how to access the vitality secrets contained in ancient yogic knowledge so that you can sculpt your ideal body, free your inner self, and transform your life with yoga and pilates.

We make hundreds of decisions every day about our lives. These decisions are all based upon what we think will make us happier, or what will provide us with more of the things we tell ourselves we need to feel successful and complete.

There is a tendency to think that if we do less we will be less, but with *Yogapilates* actually producing less movement – but doing it more proficiently – nourishes and rejuvenates the body and mind, while also strengthening and toning the muscles and the internal organs.

Yogapilates takes you through step-by-step movements to explore your own body with yoga and pilates without losing the purity of either form. Once you have mastered the individual techniques, you can then fit the sequences at the back of the book to fit comfortably into your everyday life. The results should make you become stronger and more toned, shift any excess weight, ease back pain, or simply re-address your posture.

A varied approach with the same aim

Although yoga and pilates originated and developed from vastly different philosophies, they share one overriding benefit – both open up a holistic journey to a healthier lifestyle.

Similarities between yoga and pilates

Neither form of exercise is competitive, and both encourage a social approach to movement. Pilates is more social than yoga as there is more interaction between the students and teacher on a more casual level. Yoga, however, has an inward focus, where it is common for students not to speak before and after practice to maintain the internalization of the meditations.

Beginners also tend to find yoga and pilates less intimidating than the traditional "gym scene" of mind-numbing weight-lifting and automated machines.

Physiologically, both yoga and pilates work from the inside out, which also sets them apart from other training methods. Controlled breathing in both forms is especially important as it relates to the nervous system. The quietening of the nervous system begins as the breath naturally slows down through the movements and breath-related dynamics.

You will see in your practice sections later in the book that every movement has a breath instruction. It is exactly this synchronization of breath and body dynamic that releases your body from the "fight or flight" response of the stress hormones. Your heart rate slows, your blood pressure lowers, and your body becomes more open and fluid.

Origin to insertion

Yoga and pilates both work muscles from origin to insertion, which means that you get the full range of body motion through the movement patterns. You will develop slim and elongated muscles that produce long and lean lines. Both practices are also notable for encouraging balance, strong posture, coordination, and flexibility or strength to help realign and strengthen the body for an energetic lifestyle.

Yogapilates teaches you the obvious similarities and the contrasting approaches that are necessary to achieve your mind and body goals. This book is not a fusion programme showing you how to combine yoga and pilates, but a valuable tool to help you understand the clear differences, so you can do the exercises with understanding. We have maintained the integrity of yoga and pilates in their unique and very separate forms, so you may feel and experience the subtle changes.

You will not be performing dangerous back bends or sitting and meditating for hours – these are not realistic practices, physically or psychologically, for our busy contemporary world.

The benefits of the programme

The transformations that you can expect from this programme are wide and varied, and depend on the individual, but the following are all proven outcomes that have been experienced by thousands of students:

* The shedding of unwanted weight
* Strong, sculpted, and lean muscles
* An inner oasis of calm and composure, even in the midst of everyday pressures
* Stress-busting strategies achieved through meditation
* Focused mental clarity
* The ability to catnap
* Back-care remedies
* The ability to walk taller and with head-turning confidence
* Greater mental alertness and energy levels
* Better skin and hair health
* Stronger immune system

The synergy – East meets West

It is easy to miss the unique qualities of yoga and pilates as separate forms in a world where gyms and health clubs offer fusion programmes where the two forms are mixed and diluted in order to provide a "fun performance workout".

This has happened mainly through lack of time, resulting in students who do not take on board the real objective of these concepts and just opt for the ambitious body-shaping and physical results. Although these programmes have their place in introducing new students into the mind and body arena, they can also misinterpret the pure objective of the internal rewards of pure pilates and pure yoga, which greatly assist the outer physical benefits.

Ayurvedic and western medicine

Eastern holistic healing, such as spiritual healing or Ayurvedic medicine, has worked very well, with supervision, alongside conventional Western medicine to combat illness and disease. The same principle applies when practising yoga, an eastern form of holistic healing, with the equally successful western elements of postural and core strength introduced by Joseph Pilates in his programme.

The distinctive practices of these two exercise forms can be combined to nourish and rejuvenate the human body and mind, encouraging the practitioner to stay young and energetic. *Yogapilates* teaches you elements of both practices to give you an awareness of what works for your body so that you can make your own intelligent choices.

what is yoga?

Yoga is an age-old mix of spiritual awareness and physical movement that was developed in India around 5000 years ago. Yoga is the union of the breath and body, and our body, mind, and spirit. It has become so successful because of its therapeutic effects not only on the physical body but on the internal body systems, the mind, and spirit.

Yoga origins

It is difficult to give a short history of yoga as there are so many different types. It is one of the six orthodox systems of Indian philosophy, collated and systemized by Patanjali in his classical work the *Yoga Sutras*. This collection of sayings was written around 200–400 BC and they give the eight-step path of yoga detailing a code of behaviour, which, if followed in all its elements, allows you to experience everlasting happiness and freedom from suffering.

It is useful to look at the following two key quotations to gain more understanding of the origins and purpose of yoga:

"As a diamond has many different facets reflecting various prisms of light, so does the word yoga. Each facet producing varying shades of colours, which can be aspects of the entire complex range of human desire to harness inner peace, health, and happiness."
B. K. S. Iyengar

In layman's terms: The meaning of this quotation will not become apparent until you begin to practise yoga, and as a result start to unveil the tensions and fears that exist inside you. When you are practising yoga regularly and with sensitivity, the movements may be experienced as if you are "making shapes in space" on a purely physical plane. Achieving a higher mental, emotional, and spiritual state will follow in time.

As you practise yoga, your body and mind will throw you varying degrees of resistance and obstacles, but try to work with these every time you perform the postures and see how gradually you work through these barriers to achieve more benefits from each different pose.

The Kathopanishad

The story of Kathopanishad describes yoga as:

"when the senses are stilled, when the mind is at rest, when the intellect wavers not – then, say the wise, the highest stage is reached. This steady control of the senses and mind has been defined as yoga. He who attains it is free from delusion."

In laymans terms: With the increase in unhealthy diets, smoking and drinking, and a pressurized 24-hour lifestyle, it is no wonder that we are getting fatter, our breathing rate is increasing, and our heart and lungs are becoming blocked.

The advice shown here is to slow down and allow your senses to quieten. This happens with an awareness of the breathing process and achieving sensitivity with your body. Stop trying to do more, as all you are doing is creating stress, the biggest cause of illness or disease in the modern world. There has never been a better time to reap the rewards of this age-old philosophy of Eastern healing – to calm the senses and clear your ever-busy mind.

Openness

Yoga practice has lasted so long and is in such demand, simply because it is good for your body, mind, and spirit, and it enhances your life. It is a comprehensive discipline, and although it works your body physically, it also has beneficial effects on the mind and emotions. Basically, yoga is the organized stretching of the body that is undertaken regularly and in a systematic way. When you practise yoga, you begin to open your joints and lengthen your muscles, and this creates space within your own body.

Then, by combining yoga breathing with the poses you also receive the therapeutic effects of a calmer nervous system. Yoga teaches you to become more comfortable with your body and to control your mind. This is the secret of yoga: it is not about becoming a better and different person, it is about being happy with who you are.

Benefits

Yoga calms the nervous system, supports the immune system, and allows the internal organs to work more efficiently – people who practise yoga often look younger than they really are. Your body will feel longer, leaner, and stronger as your body and mind sensitivity is increased through this harmonious practice. It is no surprise that yoga has lasted

thousands of years and that its popularity is increasing as it is an exercise discipline that has something for everyone. It exercises every single muscle in the body, and tones and invigorates the organs. It also detoxifies the body as the movements increase blood flow and encourage the removal of waste products. There is an added cosmetic effect of better blood circulation as your skin tone improves and acquires a characteristic radiancy. People who practise yoga regularly also tend to avoid the stiffening of the joints and muscles that other people suffer in later life.

One of the best effects of yoga practice is that it generates more energy, making you feel fitter and healthier, and giving you an overall feeling of well-being.

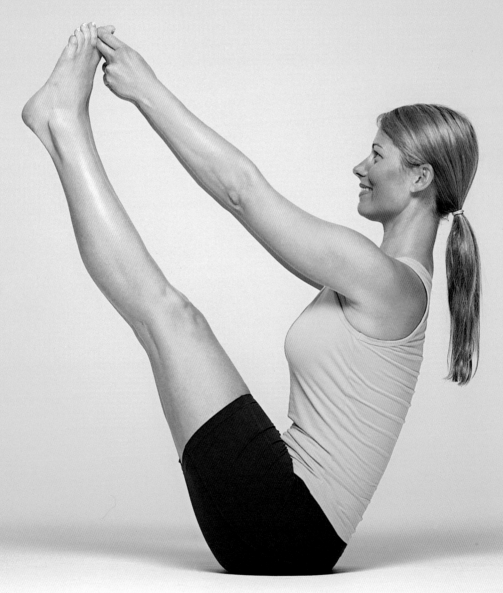

Styles of Hatha Yoga

Many styles and schools of yoga are available. They all include Hatha Yoga, a discipline thought to have begun around the year 1000 and the first to combine physical exercises and deep breathing to help concentrate the mind for meditation. The varying styles and approaches to Hatha Yoga are listed below.

Iyengar Yoga

Introduced by B. K. S. Iyengar in India in the mid-twentieth century, this form of yoga emphasizes alignment in posture (asana) particularly in the standing poses, and gives an understanding of how the body is structured. It is a safe form of yoga to practise, respecting the laws of structural anatomy, physiology, and internal energetics, but can sometimes neglect the vinyasas (the transient fluidity of movements in-between postures, see p.30) and bandhas (body harnesses, see p.31). However, its focus on alignment is its vital key, and Iyengar was also the first person to introduce yoga belts and blocks for use by beginners to the practice.

Ashtanga Vinyasa Yoga

This is a presentation of classical Hatha Yoga, developed in the twentieth century by Pattabhi Jois who learnt the form from its originator, the eighteenth-century scholar Krishnamacharya. It is based upon the ancient Sanskrit text the *Yoga Kurunta*, which Krishnamacharya adapted for the modern world. It commonly over-emphasizes one or more aspects of yoga practice at the expense of others. This may be fluidity and strength at the expense of sensitivity and alignment, or too much power at the expense of sensitivity. This sometimes results in body imbalance and does not represent the complete yoga system.

Viniyoga

Taught by T. K. V. Desikachar in Madras, this style of yoga uses step-by-step movement progression (vinyasa krama) using the breath as the guide. It focuses on individual needs and includes asanas, chanting, pranayama, and meditation, but sometimes neglects the subtleties of alignment and bandhas (see p.31).

Dynamic Yoga

Developed by Godfrey Devereux in the latter part of the twentieth century, Dynamic Yoga is the safe vinyasa krama progression to the more traditional Ashtanga Vinyasa Yoga. It clarifies the technical aspects of Hatha Yoga, integrating them all in the classical way but in a modified format. It unifies the teaching methods of Hatha Yoga, Ashtanga Yoga, Power Yoga, and Viniyoga. Dynamic Yoga encourages a soft and gradual entry to the inner self through safe, progressing postures.

Modern yoga

When we consider that yoga originated in India around 5000 years ago, we have to measure yoga today against the very different climate and stresses that were evident at this time. India is a much warmer climate than Europe and originally the yogis were able to devote six to eight hours of their day mastering the art of yoga, seeking enlightenment away from the material aspects of life.

Fitness Yoga – shapemaking

In general terms, the western world has a colder climate, people have less available time, and are exposed to high levels of stress. This has resulted in something I call "Fitness Yoga" being mistaken for pure yoga. In truth, demand has exceeded the amount of experienced yoga teachers available.

In Fitness Yoga, similar shapes to the yoga postures are performed quickly so that the emphasis is on the physical rather than the mental. In fact, the view is that the faster the postures are performed, the more can be done. This is not pure yoga. For maximum benefit yoga should be performed with the mental and physical approaches in balance.

Body heat

One of the obvious effects of performing continuous movements is the build up of physical heat. As the body's ligaments, muscles, and joints warm up, they soften and open and we start to sweat. If the body experiences long periods of sweating, then we have to use up more heat to replace it. Sweat should act as a thermal layer like a wetsuit; therefore sweat should not be wiped away as it will use up excess energy and tire us. The heat coming from yoga practice should be felt as an internal subtle and constant flow, not the same external burning or draining heat that is felt in the hot sun, for example.

Ullolas and vinyasas

The yoga practices shown here advise longer breathing exercises called ullolas, which are simple breathing exercises that unite the breath (see p.37) and a fluidity of movement called vinyasa to ensure essential joint and muscle opening takes place before starting the main programme (see p.30).

Relaxation

Advice is also given on the importance of a nourishing, long rest and relaxation at the end of yoga practice to allow time for reflection, and to offset lethargy or fatigue (see p.80). Above all effective yoga practice will result in the stilling of the busy mind to encourage the ultimate healing state, inner calm and rejuvenation.

A reluctance to practise

When you first practise yoga, you will find yourself thinking of the million and one other things you need to do, but with concentration and discipline you will begin to enjoy your session, and feel your body opening and softening. This will not always be a pleasant journey as you may have many years of resistance from slouching, lack of physical activity, or doing too much wrong exercise. This will disappear as you practise yoga; you will see how much more supple and toned you are, and how much calmer you feel.

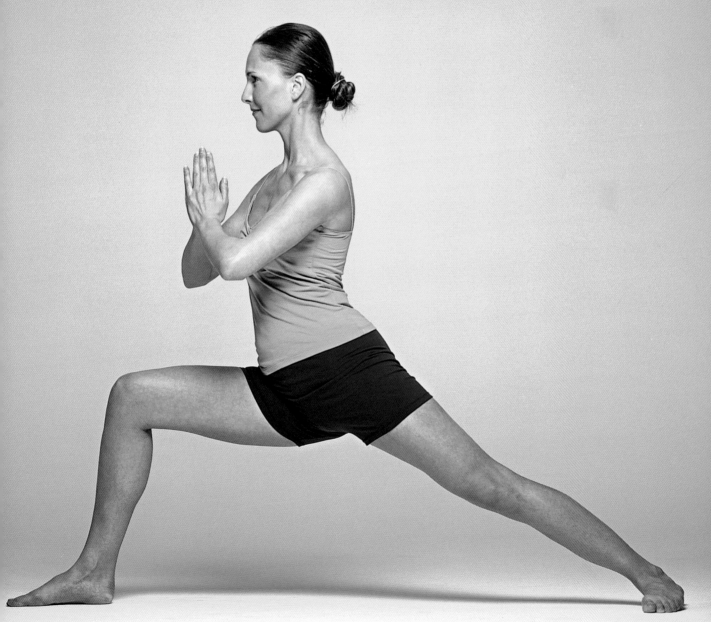

what is pilates?

Pilates is a unique programme that was devised by Joseph Hubertus Pilates in the 1920s. He conceived it so that dancers could improve their technique, but it soon became a popular exercise method. The movements create lean, strong muscles, improve balance and circulation, and give increased confidence.

Pilates origins

Joseph Pilates was born in 1880 into a world that had recently discovered that good or bad postural habits affected people's overall health. Born near the north German city of Düsseldorf, he grew up a frail, sickly child. The worry of developing tuberculosis is thought to have inspired him to work hard at improving his health and physical fitness. By the age of 14 he had become so fit that he was posing as a model for anatomical drawings.

Pilates became a keen gymnast, skier, and diver. He is believed to have worked in Britain from 1912–14 as a circus performer, boxer, and a self-defence instructor. During World War I (1914–18) he was interned in England as a German national, and he developed his fitness skills by teaching them to fellow internees. He started to gain widespread respect in his field, particularly when none of his internees practising his programme became ill during a bad war-time flu epidemic. About a year after his return to Germany after the war, Pilates is said to have influenced Rudolph Von Laban, the originator of the widely used system of dance notation. Soon after, in 1923, Pilates emigrated to the USA and settled in New York.

In his new country Pilates opened his own studio. He produced a booklet called *Your Health* which showed some of the exercise apparatus that had become a hallmark of his system. By 1939 his exercise regime was a renowned success, and Pilates was able to boast a vast client list, from writers such as Christopher Isherwood to well-known dancers from the New York City Ballet.

Over the years he refined his exercise methods and in 1945 published a list of core exercises called "Return to Life through Contrology." The exercises formed the basis of a self-help fitness method for preventing degenerative illnesses, improving body tone and shape, and increasing longevity.

Modern pilates

Joseph Pilates always wanted his exercises to be a fitness aid for everyone, but it was only after his death that they spread beyond the domain of performers and dancers.

Pilates is now one of the most successful movement programmes, as it offers effective solutions to anyone of any age who is keen to stay in shape. The success of the programme has produced a pilates-based exercise method which, having responded to new scientific discoveries about how the brain and body interact, is taking structural fitness and body balance into the twenty-first century.

Joseph Pilates was looking to stretch the body to the full to bring maximum benefit to the person exercising. Even a trained athlete would have difficulty in performing some of the original movements he devised. This is because they use a refined level of muscle control and a coordination with which few of us are familiar.

The art of balance

Most exercise programmes lack one basic ingredient: balance. While weight training, for example, maximizes muscular strength, and aerobics increases overall stamina, Pilates exercises focus on balancing the actions of the body's whole structure: the skeleton, the joints, the muscles, and the major organs. Pilates was critical of the flat feet and curved spines that he saw around him, identified by him as the postural defects caused by using poorly designed furniture, and the unbalanced exercises promoted by other physical trainers, which he felt distorted the body.

The association between physical and mental well-being was Joseph Pilates' guiding principle, and modern pilates still aims at achieving the coordination of body and mind through practising exercise movements.

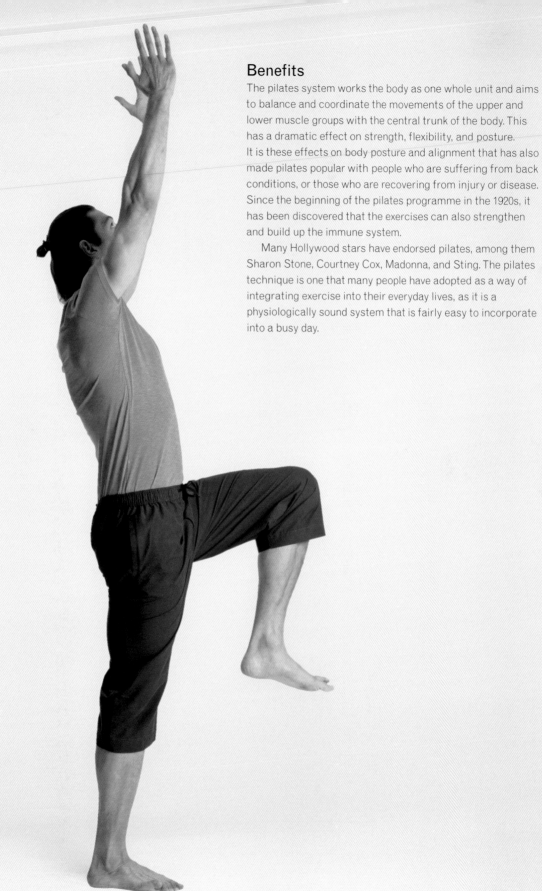

Benefits

The pilates system works the body as one whole unit and aims to balance and coordinate the movements of the upper and lower muscle groups with the central trunk of the body. This has a dramatic effect on strength, flexibility, and posture.

It is these effects on body posture and alignment that has also made pilates popular with people who are suffering from back conditions, or those who are recovering from injury or disease. Since the beginning of the pilates programme in the 1920s, it has been discovered that the exercises can also strengthen and build up the immune system.

Many Hollywood stars have endorsed pilates, among them Sharon Stone, Courtney Cox, Madonna, and Sting. The pilates technique is one that many people have adopted as a way of integrating exercise into their everyday lives, as it is a physiologically sound system that is fairly easy to incorporate into a busy day.

core basics

The "core" of the body is the central foundation for both yoga and pilates and consists of the brain, eyes, ears, jaw, palate, throat, abdomen, spine, pelvis, and associative connective tissues. Having an understanding of the important muscles in your body, how they work, and their role, will give you a greater understanding of your body structure.

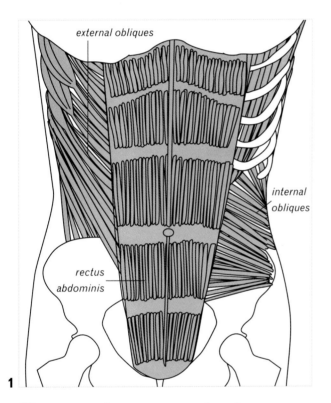

external obliques

internal obliques

rectus abdominis

1

POSTURE

Many different movements can cause postural problems. For example a child walking to school carrying a heavy bag on their back is forced to lean forwards, placing stress on the lumbar spine and shortening the hips. Ballet dancers often walk with their feet turned out, which creates a shortening of the outside muscles of the legs.

Even earlier in life, toddlers who walk around in thick nappies develop abnormal walking movements. In adult life, jobs such as gardening, laying paving, or carrying a baby on one hip can cause the back to curve forward or distort the shape of the lower spine, leading to chronic backache.

Posture is the foundation of alignment in any good yoga or pilates practice. In these disciplines emphasis is placed upon how the pelvis and trunk muscles work in relation to the rest of the body. The trunk, abdomen, spine, and pelvis are like the chassis of your car – if any part becomes unbalanced or injured the whole vehicle (body) becomes misaligned. Wear and tear on the joints and muscles becomes obvious and causes discomfort.

The muscles you need to know

▲ Rectus abdominis and obliques

The abdomen has four large muscles wrapped around the abdomen like a corset. These muscles support and cushion the internal organs, holding them in place. The rectus abdominis (R.A.) is commonly known as the "six pack" when developed. The muscles lie very close to the surface of the skin, which is why you can see them when they are toned. These muscles flex the trunk, pulling the lower body towards the rib cage. Tightening the abdominal muscles with sit-up exercises creates pressure in the R.A., which in time can deepen the lower back curve. When these muscles are strong and elastic they maintain good posture by keeping the lower back curve shallow and the pelvis correctly aligned. The external obliques (E.O.) travel from the ribs to the pubic bone and wrap around the sides of the abdomen. They work with the smaller internal obliques (I.O.) beneath them, and with the R.A., to flex or bend the trunk. The obliques are also used for lateral balance.

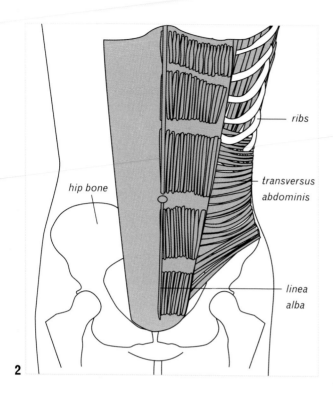
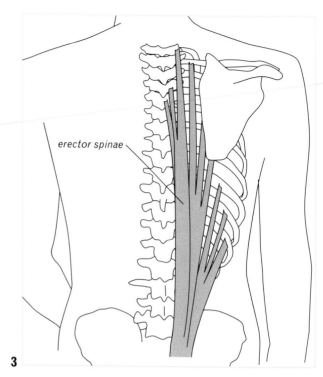

2

3

▲ Transversus abdominis

The transversus abdominis (T.A.) muscles lie beneath the rectus abdominis and internal obliques. Their fibres run in a cross direction to the abdomen, creating strength in the area. The muscles originate in the lower six ribs and the top of the hip bone and stretch into the linea alba (a strip of connective tissue, see diagram 2). The T.A. prevents the pelvic floor from sagging (see diagram 5). Structural integrity and balance depends upon maintaining tone and elasticity in these important muscle groups. The T.A. is much more important than the R.A. for bringing about true core strength and correct pelvic alignment.

▶ Rotatores spinae

The rotator muscles help rotate the body from side to side. They work in tandem with the multifidus, or spine, muscles. Both sets of rotators and multifidus muscles on either side of the spine work together to stretch the whole trunk. For example, the muscles on the left side work to rotate the trunk to the right and vice versa.

▲ Erector spinae

The spine has over 100 pairs of muscles supporting it that allow it to flex, extend, and rotate in all directions. The erector spinae muscles support the vertebrae that make up the spine and keep them firmly held in position. Working together they lift the trunk and flex and rotate the spine. With the synergy of strong T.A. muscles you offset any existing body weakness, and maintain the good posture and alignment of upper and lower body stability.

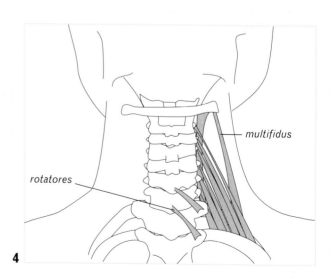

4

THE PELVIC FLOOR

The pelvis cradles the abdominal organs. The pelvic floor is a hammock-shaped muscle that runs from the front pubic bone to the tailbone at the back. If the muscle weakens and sags, the abdomen protrudes and the other muscles of the bladder, rectum, and vagina in women, become stressed and lose tone.

Your pelvic floor is such an important body structure that if you let it lose tone you can throw your whole body out of alignment. Your can lose your pelvic tilt, your posture will sag, your abdomen domes and protrudes, and your urogenital muscles weaken.

It is hard to find your pelvic floor muscles as they are invisible and also plagued by taboos relating to sexuality. Strong pelvic floor muscles and internal lifting exercises in this area have been proven to strengthen abdomen stability and increase spine support through the pioneering work of Dr Arnold Kegel in the 1960s.

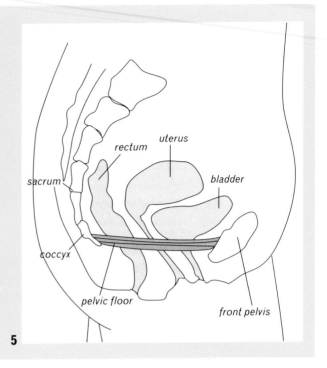

5

Pelvic floor movements in yoga and pilates

Eventually you will learn to refine your pelvic floor technique and keep the front part engaged to 20–30 per cent for all pilates movements as a basic part of the exercise.

In yoga as your breathing deepens on the exhalation, the diaphragm relaxes but you learn to keep the intercostal muscles between the ribs engaged to keep the rib cage broad. Towards the end of a series of emptying out breaths, the outer muscles of the abdomen contract, squeezing more air from the lungs. This assists in emptying the pubic abdomen of all breath and a gentle natural lift of the perineum will draw the pelvic floor upwards.

In pilates this movement is activated as an initiated instruction, but in yoga it happens naturally as your diaphragm relaxes and your lower abdomen muscles flatten towards the spine. This pelvic floor contraction helps to stabilize the pelvis and provides a safe and strong foundation from which to hold the more challenging yoga postures, or to simply tone the abdomen or strengthen the spine in pilates (see bandhas p.31).

Keeping pelvic floor muscles strong

If you work and lift your pelvic floor muscles as you exercise, it protects your lower spine and stops your abdomen from straining when you lift heavy objects.

The pelvic floor muscles function best when the pelvis is centred (see diagram 5). The abdominal organs should fit into the centre space and be nicely balanced.

If the muscles of the pelvic floor become weak and go slack, they can no longer support the abdominal organs, which then start to sag and eventually collapse or fall through the base of the pelvic girdle – this in turn puts immense stress on the lumbar, or lower spine.

Contracting and lifting the pelvic floor

As the pelvic floor contracts, the muscles that move the ribs also contract, preventing them from moving, so in turn the chest cannot expand and the abdominal muscles tighten. Therefore if you hold your pelvic floor tightly you will restrict breathing, movement, and speech, so it should be gently lifted – try only about 20–30 per cent lifting pressure as a strengthening exercise, and then release.

As you become stronger, you can maintain the lift for a bit longer. As you learn to exhale and draw the abdominal muscles inwards, the pelvic floor will engage and lift. You should not hollow the abdomen in and lift the pelvic floor together. One technique at a time is enough to involve these important muscles without causing any strain.

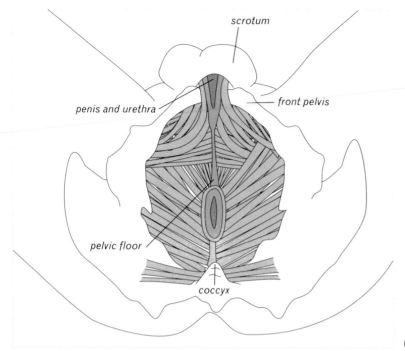

scrotum

penis and urethra

front pelvis

pelvic floor

coccyx

◄ Male pelvic floor

Men can do pelvic floor exercises just as well as women. They can partially feel the lift through the perineum, a similar feeling to trying to stop yourself from emptying your bladder. You can become sensitive to which muscles to move by performing certain exercises (see p.51).

In men the pelvic floor surrounds the anus and penis. The coccygeus is the most important of the range of outer muscles in the diaphragm of pelvic floor muscles. The pelvic floor is funnel shaped, so any pressure on it is directed downwards. The pelvic floor muscles surround the external sex organs in men (see diagram 6) and the vagina in women (see diagram 7).

6

► Female pelvic floor

When the pelvic floor muscles are viewed from below, they make a figure eight with the perineum in the centre. The loops are formed by the sphincter muscles around the anus, sex organs, and bladder. Both men and women tighten and relax these muscles when emptying or holding on from emptying the bladder. Women have the ability to tighten or engage the muscle that surrounds the vagina, while men use the corresponding muscle to control erection and ejaculation.

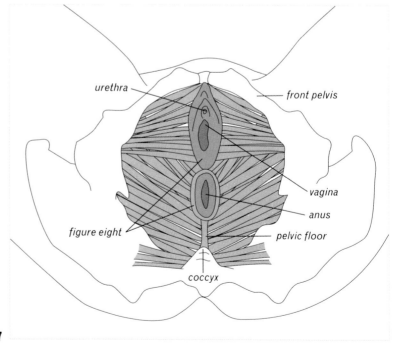

urethra

front pelvis

vagina

anus

pelvic floor

figure eight

coccyx

7

preparation

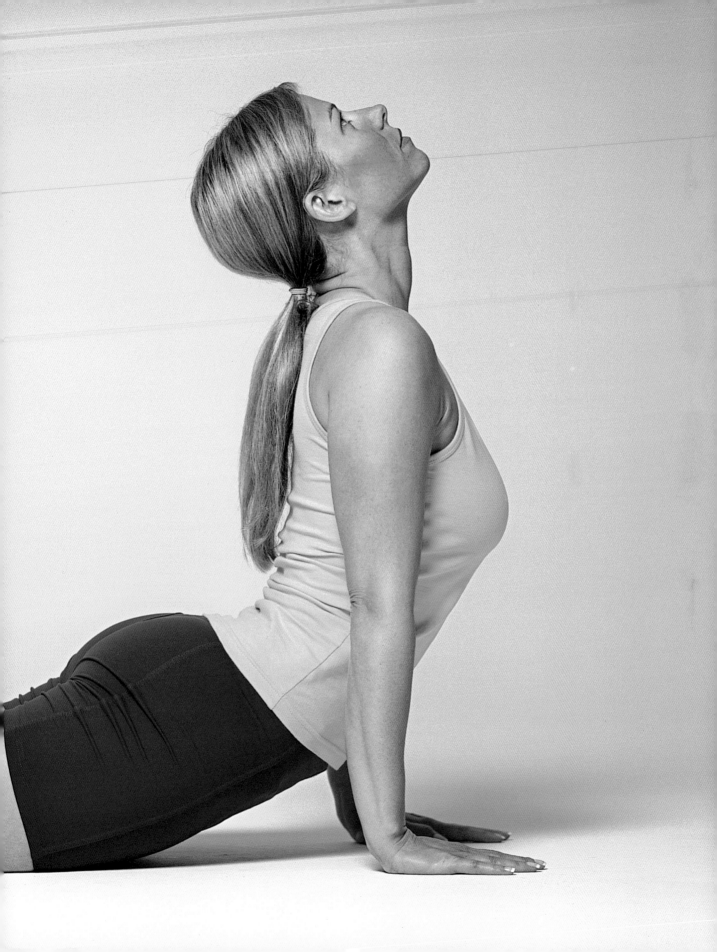

pilates path secrets and techniques

The eight principles of pilates practice

Pilates uses eight main principles that help you to master and refine your technique. Each principle below will challenge you in a different way, and it is the harmonious relationship between all of them that gives you the best results.

Concentration

Pilates is a mental (neuro) and physical (muscular) programme that trains both body and mind. As you relax your body you become more focused and more aware. When you do the exercises in this book you will need to focus your attention on refining each movement that you make, using the sensory feedback your mind and body receives.

The techniques will need to be repeated and experienced in various situations for them to be refined and tuned like a musical instrument. Eventually the movements will become automatic but you will still have to concentrate because there is always a further level of tuning to achieve. This body tuning can then be applied to, and improve, other daily activities.

Relaxation

This is the starting point for everyone learning pilates. Beginning with relaxation ensures that everyday stress is not brought into a session. Learning how to recognize and release unwanted tension is essential before you work out, as it helps to prevent the use of the wrong muscles. Pilates will teach you how to switch off over-dominant muscles that can otherwise overwork, using unsound movement patterns.

Areas of common tension are the brain and the pelvic floor. These are the top and bottom parts of your nervous system, which is housed by the spinal column. Most people also hold tension in the backs of their shoulders and the neck. Also, if you sit for long periods the muscles around the thighs, lumbar spine, hips, and hamstrings become too tight. The Relaxation Pose (see p.81) is the best place to start and finish most pilates and yoga practice sessions. The term "relaxation" does not mean falling asleep or collapsing, but a position where unnecessary tension is released before movement.

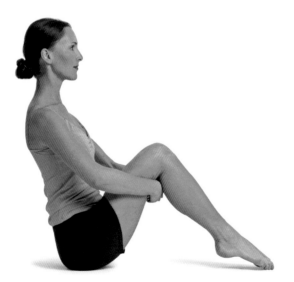

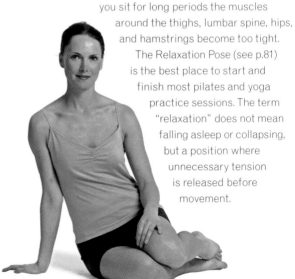

Coordination

As you move through the sections in this book, you will gradually be able to add movements such as rotation, flexion, and extension to the basic understanding and body tuning you have initially achieved, at the same time as maintaining your strong centre or neutral spine.

With practice the coordination of these progressions improves your muscle memory. The actual process of learning this coordination is excellent mental and physical training, encouraging the brain to remember positive and useful movement patterns. Try to start with smaller motions and then build up to more complicated ones.

The movements must be performed correctly and with honesty otherwise you will feed the brain incorrect data. Just like a computer programme, the brain will be programmed according to the feedback your body gives it.

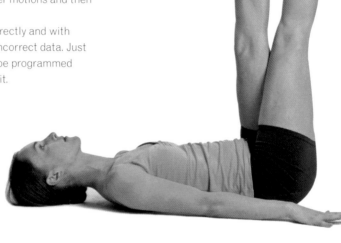

Alignment

In pilates we are constantly reminding the body of how it should be utilizing the correct muscle groups to sit, stand, and move correctly to rectify any imbalances. If you exercise without paying attention to the correct position of the joints, you risk stressing them, while also building imbalance in the surrounding muscle groups. The pelvic and lumbar stability exercises (see pp.32–3) help you to find correct neutral alignment. This is the position where the spine and its discs are under minimal stress or compression. You should practise finding your neutral alignment in several different positions: lying, sitting, and standing, and also use it during the coordination of movement.

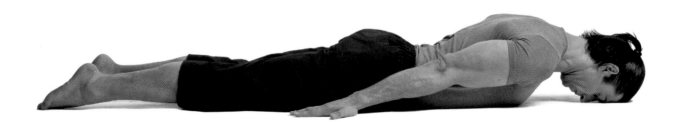

Breathing

Most of us breathe inefficiently. Ideally we should breathe fully and deeply into the back and sides of the lungs. This is logical because the lungs are situated in the rib cage and by expanding them front, back, and sides, the volume of the cavity is increased and the capacity for oxygen intake is higher. Breathing deeply also encourages maximum use of the lower part of the lungs (see Thoracic breathing p.35).

Every single pilates movement has a specific breath instruction. This enhances effective muscle use by correct breathing and timing of the breath. Generally the exertion of the movement is performed with an exhalation. Moving during the exhalation also enables you to relax into the stretch and prevents you from tensing. It also offers great stability at the hardest part of any movement and prevents you from holding your breath, which can lead to stress.

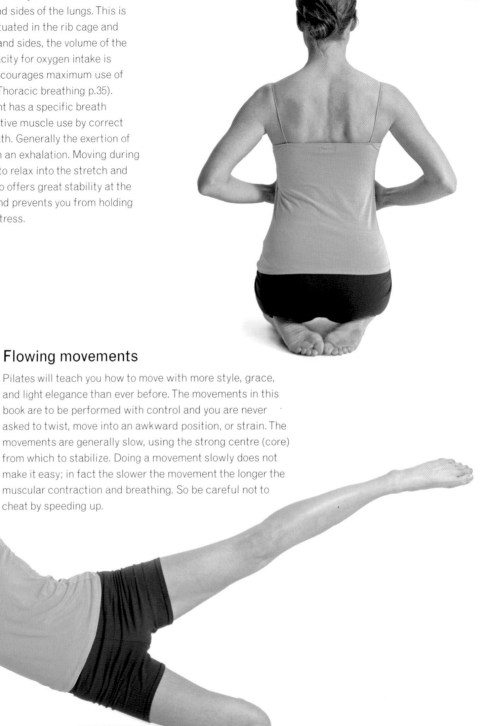

Flowing movements

Pilates will teach you how to move with more style, grace, and light elegance than ever before. The movements in this book are to be performed with control and you are never asked to twist, move into an awkward position, or strain. The movements are generally slow, using the strong centre (core) from which to stabilize. Doing a movement slowly does not make it easy; in fact the slower the movement the longer the muscular contraction and breathing. So be careful not to cheat by speeding up.

Centring

If you stand upright and hollow your navel towards your spine, your lower back will feel protected in a similar way to a corset. This was the discovery of Joseph Pilates. He had no knowledge of core stability or the multifidus/transversus abdominal muscles in the nineteenth century, but he had superb body awareness. This is why this instruction "navel to spine" filters into all pilates movements. This method has been known to sometimes inhibit breathing if it is applied too aggressively. However modern research, mostly by Arnold Kegel in 1968, publicised the importance of also utilizing the muscles of the pelvic floor for maximum stability. As you breathe out, draw up the muscles of the pelvic floor (20–30 per cent only) and hollow your abdominals back to your spine. Then hold the engagement and breathe normally. This method has immensely beneficial affects on all posture types for improving balance, stability, and mental well-being.

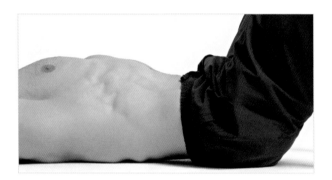
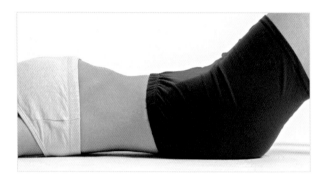

Stamina

To improve muscular strength and tone you will need to build endurance and stamina in the body. The exercises in this book will challenge your ability to maintain a neutral spine and pelvic floor engagement with various intensities. Some of the movements will offer you a harder or easier option to progress gradually. Sitting in a office all day can make you lethargic, simply because sitting poorly is tiring. The negative effects are that:

* The hamstrings and spine tighten
* The back slouches
* The rib cage compresses
* The lungs contract

This book will teach you to open and lengthen your body as your breathing becomes more efficient and you learn to relax. All pilates movements encourage the respiratory, lymphatic, and circulatory systems to function more effectively.

When your technique improves, the muscles in your back and abdomen will begin to work correctly again, and you will discover how this dramatically improves your overall stamina. You will no longer waste energy on holding onto unwanted tension or moving inefficiently.

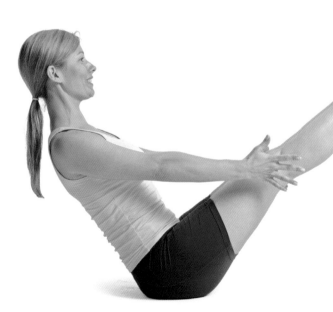

yoga path secrets and techniques

The eightfold path of Yoga as found in Patanjali's *Yoga Sutras* (c.200–400 BC) is an eight-step guide to self-realization and enlightenment. The five principles detailed on the following pages are a less detailed explanation of the eightfold path.

It is no surprise that Patanjali spoke about honesty and quality of awareness before beginning asana (posture) work, and it is these particular elements that will help you to overcome your physical or emotional obstacles or any resistance to practise.

Yoga is not about becoming flexible or strong – Patanjali intended yoga to be soft and fulfilling. Bear this in mind when you start to practise, and eradicate any pre-conceptions about what you are trying to achieve. Only then will the true rewards of this technique shine through.

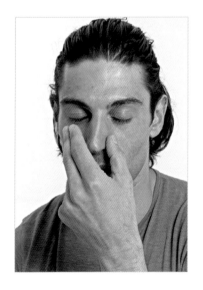

Pranayama

This approach can be compared to pilates breathing and stamina. It can be translated as "pranic capacity" or "control of the prana." Prana is energy and is therefore the breath. When prana enters the body during yoga practice the body feels completely charged with energy. When prana leaves the body, death occurs.

Prana = Energy/Breath
Yama = Discipline

Deep, conscious breathing and full expansion of the lungs is a powerful energizing tool. As more oxygen is distributed to the body's tissues, every cellular process is enhanced to aid the activity of the cells to repair, digest, detoxify, and combat disease. Nourished cells make up a healthy body and mind.

Drushti

Simply speaking, drushti is your sensitive awareness to whatever you are doing. It can be compared to concentration and breathing in pilates. Wherever else our attention is held, it must always encompass the core of our body. This includes the eyes, ears, and tongue, the front and back spine, the interior spine, the pelvic floor, and the navel.

Some yogis refer to drushti as meditation but you do not have to be still to be focused on what is actually happening. To be completely present with what is happening is drushti, even to the point where you are not thinking of anything else while you practise, even about what you are doing. Experience and feel the movement, rather than just performing it.

Generally we think before we act, then think again and refine our actions. But eventually you will learn to separate these two processes so that you may act with precision and clarity without having to think. Through practice we can learn to trust the intelligence of the body and will be able to dispense with the thinking process more easily. This is when yoga becomes meditation through action.

We must also feel the impact of the functioning body, breath, and mind from the action. We can use this feedback to refine movements further and make adjustments.

Drushti through yoga practice is a good skill to quieten the mind from stress. It will help you to slow down, calm the breath, and enjoy every moment.

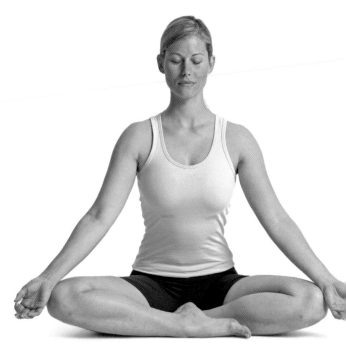

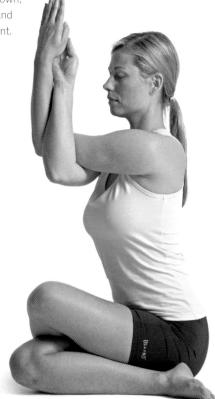

Asana

This is the structural integrity of the postures and can be compared to centring and alignment in pilates. There is so much more to asana than a simple shape in space. What is happening on the inside of the dynamic of the body is more important. It is alignment that gives the body stability and elegance. It is using the body's ability to restructure the anatomical body to bring about realignment and balance.

Asana = Posture

The basic purpose of alignment is to harmonize the body, and this does not necessarily mean achieving physical perfection. More importantly it involves harmonizing opposing lines of force to bring about structural stability. Eventually, through repetitive alignment and refining, tension is drawn out from the body cells and these new lines of force establish deeper structural integrity.

Of all the yoga postures the most important for awakening somatic intelligence and harmonizing balance are the vinyasas (see p.40) and standing postures (see pp.60–62). This is because each standing posture demands activity in every part of the body to stay stable and upright: there are no areas of inert passivity. This is why each of the classical yoga series begins with a sequence of standing poses and vinyasa.

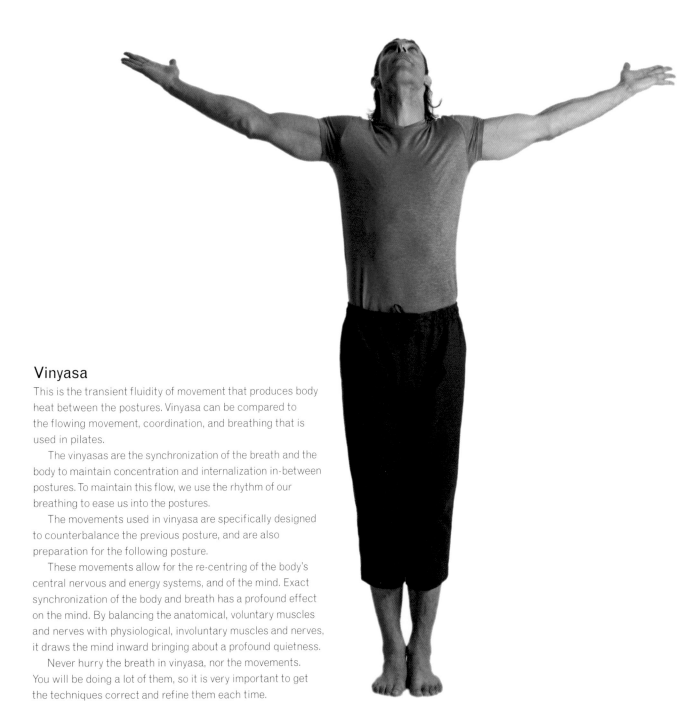

Vinyasa

This is the transient fluidity of movement that produces body heat between the postures. Vinyasa can be compared to the flowing movement, coordination, and breathing that is used in pilates.

The vinyasas are the synchronization of the breath and the body to maintain concentration and internalization in-between postures. To maintain this flow, we use the rhythm of our breathing to ease us into the postures.

The movements used in vinyasa are specifically designed to counterbalance the previous posture, and are also preparation for the following posture.

These movements allow for the re-centring of the body's central nervous and energy systems, and of the mind. Exact synchronization of the body and breath has a profound effect on the mind. By balancing the anatomical, voluntary muscles and nerves with physiological, involuntary muscles and nerves, it draws the mind inward bringing about a profound quietness.

Never hurry the breath in vinyasa, nor the movements. You will be doing a lot of them, so it is very important to get the techniques correct and refine them each time.

Bandhas

The bandhas are the core of yoga practice and can be compared to centring, breathing, and stamina in pilates. The bandhas involve the subtle muscular adjustments in the trunk related to the physiological rather than anatomical body. They use our involuntary muscles more than voluntary ones, or at least the approach is involuntary.

The breath is connected to the mind. If you suddenly remember on a plane that you have left your stove on, you feel the shock of the consequences. The "fight" response of the stress hormones rushing into your bloodstream puts everything on panic alert until a solution is found. You feel your heart rate speed up and your muscles tighten. The shock of the thought physically affects your breathing, and it speeds up and becomes more shallow.

When your mind is at ease your breathing becomes slow and deep. Calming the breath quietens the mind. Conscious breathing is a bridge between your nervous system, mind, and emotions. By engaging the sacrum, lumbar, thoracic, and cervical vertebrae, the spine is aligned and its central channel opened. By stimulating the solar plexus (in the middle of your abdomen), energy is generated and transformed. By stimulating the perineum, the central nervous system is quietened and the spine is supported in asana.

There are three bandhas or harnesses in yoga:

Jalandhara bandha – This action involves the throat harness and slows down the breath, producing *ujjayi* breathing. It is commonly used in inversions where the chin is pressed onto the chest. The air passes through the throat into the palate and makes a deep rhythmic sound.

Uddiyana bandha – This movement involves pulling in and up the muscles in the solar plexus. The muscles of inhalation act in unison with the transversus abdomen to stabilize and lengthen the abdomen.

Mula bandha – This involves pulling in the perineal body and pushing the pelvic floor upwards as a reaction to emptying the pubic abdomen, drawing the sacrum inwards. This protects the lumbar spine and stabilizes the pelvis for asana.

Some yogis say that practice without the bandhas is unsafe as then there is no support for the central trunk and pelvis while practising asana. This is common to both pilates and yoga, although each discipline approaches it very differently.

Pilates = Voluntary activation to pelvic floor engagement = neutral alignment

Yoga = Involuntary activation of pelvic floor engagement = bandhas

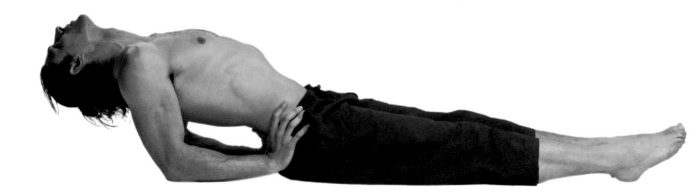

pilates and yoga alignment

This is another common thread between yoga and pilates, as both disciplines work with the natural, neutral position of the body. From the feet, through the legs and pelvis, up the trunk, to the arms, neck, and head, the stance is very similar. For correct aligned movement to take place, the body needs to be in a perfect postural alignment. The standing and lying postures are a great place to check body alignment and both of these will be referred to throughout.

Pilates alignment

What makes pilates so unique and effective for abdominal and spinal strength is the ability to stabilize your own pelvis by understanding the relationship of the transversus abdominals and multifidus (spine) muscles, and maintaining a re-aligned spine for lifting and working (see p.19).

If you exercise with the pelvis and spine out of alignment, it is common to create more muscle imbalances by putting the spine under stress. In pilates we always aim to keep the spine and pelvis in a neutral position. This automatically releases the spine from stress and allows the practitioner to re-learn the free and effortless movements that the human body once did so easily.

To find your neutral pelvis and spine position, follow the movements opposite and to centre correctly see p.27.

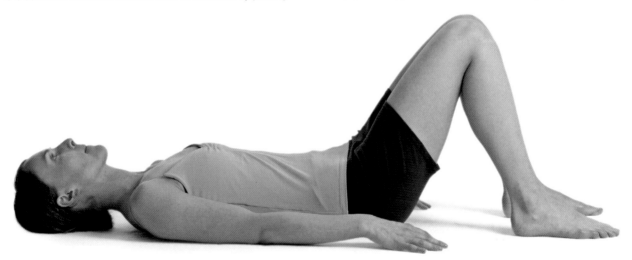

Finding the neutral position and correct breathing

These first two positions are incorrect. We will practise these first, so that you can feel the difference.

1 Pelvis in north – slouched

* Lie in the Relaxation Pose (see p.81) with your feet flat on the floor, your knees bent and your shoulders relaxed.
* Keep your head in a central position and gently inhale. As you exhale take your arms above your head in preparation for pelvis enquiry. Keep breathing normally and keep your buttocks soft.
* Imagine a compass on your lower abdomen. The navel is north and the pubic bone is south.
* Tilt your pelvis north and release your abdomen. Feel the pelvis tuck under, your waist relax and flatten and how your lower back rounds into the mat.

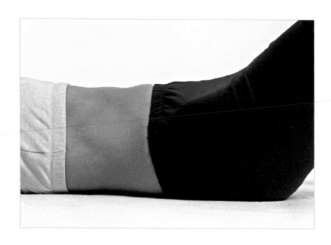

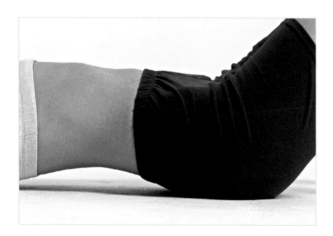

2 Pelvis in south – arched

* From the Relaxation Pose gently move your pelvis in the other direction allowing your abdomen to release so that it tilts south (do this cautiously if you have a back injury).
* Your lower back arches, your sternum and floating ribs lift, and your abdomen domes outwards.
* Slowly come back down to the relaxation position.

3 Pelvis in centre – neutral

* Lying in the Relaxation Pose, gently draw your abdomen towards your spine to hollow the core. Aim for a central position between the north and the south. This is where the back is neither arched nor rounded into the mat. Make sure your pubic bone and hip bones are level, and your sacrum sits squarely on the floor.
* Once you have found your neutral position, practise inhaling and filling out your rib cage. Feel your rib cage broaden, then exhale to gently empty the pubic abdomen as you practise stabilizing the pelvis.
* Practise 10 breaths without losing your new awareness of the neutral spine position.

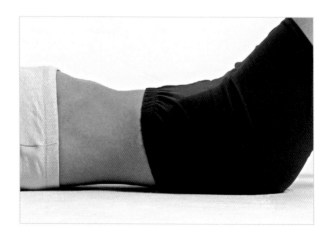

Yoga alignment

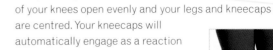

Basic standing posture

This foundation pose is a vitally important standing position. Ensure that you are distributing your weight evenly.

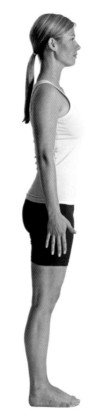

* Stand upright with your weight balanced evenly on each foot. Inhale.
* Exhale and suck thigh muscles into your thigh bones, energizing your legs.
* Inhale and lift your armpits away from your hip bones so that your chest becomes broad and full.
* Exhale and extend your arms downwards from your trunk, hands spread, keeping your shoulders down.
* Keep your palms wide with your fingertips spread.
* Looking straight ahead, keep the core of your body soft and untensed.
* Keep breathing rhythmically.

Feet

The feet balance the legs and connect to the pelvis, which stabilizes the main body weight. Check your feet are broad, full, and balanced to prevent misalignment.

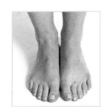

* Stand with your feet touching at the inner heel and big toes, or keep your feet parallel to each other.
* Keep your weight evenly balanced between the balls of your feet and heels.
* Maintain a close contact between your inner ankles so they do not roll apart or forwards.
* Lift up through the arches of your feet as the balls of the toes and the inner and outer heels press down.

Legs

This sealing process of the legs (and arms) is used in other positions to the one above. When sealed the legs are lifted, almost squeezed, away from the pelvis, releasing the foundation of some of their weight. It is more than an anatomical process, it is a physiological one promoting a deep release in the tissue nerves, capillaries, ducts, veins, and channels of the skin and joints. This allows a fuller and freer flow of liquids and your body's nerve impulses.

* Pull your thigh muscles into the bones so that the backs of your knees open evenly and your legs and kneecaps are centred. Your kneecaps will automatically engage as a reaction to this instruction.

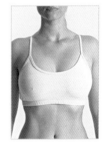

* Bring your weight forward to the balls of the front of both feet by pushing from your heels. The legs remain straight with the front thigh pulling the thighbone out of the knee joint, and the front calf lifting the shin bone out of the back knee joint.

Trunk and head

Paying attention to the position, shape, and quality of the pelvis, abdomen, chest, and neck will determine the shape and quality of your spine. We are not talking about correcting the spine so that it is "straight", as it should never be straight. The aim is for it to be fully extended with space, therefore allowing freedom of movement between each vertebra – no movement can occur if the spine is straight. Movement is seen in the curves. It takes time to realign the spine and strengthen and lengthen the relevant muscles to centre the sacrum and stabilize the pelvis and lumbar region safely. If you re-educate and develop harmony within the trunk and the rest of the body you will see the benefits.

* Stand and lift your armpits away from your hip bones, broaden your ribs, and pull in and lift up your solar plexus and upwards so your chest becomes broad, and full. Keep your abdomen long, passive and empty (see Uddiyana bandha p.31).
* Keep your pelvic floor soft, as you lift your hip bones so that they flatten and broaden. Your sacrum and perineum are lifted up, and your anus stays soft (see Mula bandha p.31).

Hands

The hands equalize the rate of oxygen into the lungs, so keep them broad and open. They form part of the foundation pose.

* Spread weight evenly over your hands.
* Broaden your hands comfortably, but do not over-stretch.
* Softly extend your hands from a broad palm.
* Keep your hands in line with your wrists.

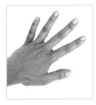

pilates breathing

The breathing techniques for both pilates and yoga are very similar in that they both use conscious awareness of breathing, unlike other forms of exercise such as aerobics or dance. Pilates breathing is controlled through the goal of strengthening the lower abdominal muscles. The exertion in a pilates movement is always performed on a breath exhalation, irrelevant of whether flexion (closing the body) or extension (opening) is used. However in yoga, an inhalation is always performed on extensions, while exhalation occurs with a flexion movement (see also bandhas on p.31 and pilates path secrets: breathing on p.26).

Most of us breathe inefficiently. All pilates movements are created to establish the connection of your breathing to emphasize the correct trunk and spine posture. The timing of the breath is crucial to the success of all pilates and yoga movements for different reasons. The breath alone can help lengthen your abdomen, broaden your chest and upper back, and train the correct muscle recruitment patterns for everyday core strength.

The ideal breathing action is to breathe in fully and deeply to the back and sides of your lungs. This is logical because the lungs are situated in the rib cage and by expanding it, the cavity increases, allowing more oxygen to be taken in.

The lungs need to open front, back, right, and left. To do this you need to train your breathing, your abdominals, and all the other muscles of inhalation and exhalation to allow for the lungs to fully open in all four directions. Most of us only open the front lungs by breathing shallowly and lightly.

This simple practice alone creates good trunk posture and increases abdominal and diaphragmatic strength.

Thoracic breathing
* Sit on your heels or stand. Wrap a wide scarf around your ribs, crossing it over at the front.
* Holding the opposite ends of the band, gently pull it tight.
* Breathe in and allow your ribs to expand the scarf, making sure that your breastbone does not lift too high. Think about breathing wide.
* As you breathe out, tighten the scarf a little to help empty your lungs fully and relax your rib cage (allow it to soften).

Repeat as many times as necessary to establish a hollow abdomen and a full rib cage with each breath.

* Note: as you practise, you will notice that on breathing out, your abdomen will hollow and your pelvic floor will engage, giving more lumbar and pelvic stability. Ultimately you will keep these muscles engaged as you breathe in and out but only ever to a maximum hold of 20–30 per cent pelvic floor engagement. Draw in your abdomen or lift your pelvic floor muscles but not both together (see pp.32–3).

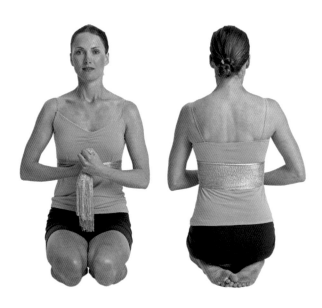

yoga breathing

Yoga breathing is essentially a free breathing that pacifies the nervous system and is synergized with all movement. No breathing is forced or controlled, whereas pilates teaches breath control. Other important differences between the two disciplines occur with the engagement of the pelvic floor when hollowing the pubic abdomen.

The yogi's life is not measured by the number of the days he lives but by the number of breaths he takes. Therefore, he always follows the proper rhythmic patterns of slow, deep breathing. These rhythmic patterns help to:

* Strengthen the respiratory system
* Pacify the nervous system
* Reduce mental or physical craving

As desires, temptations, and cravings diminish, the mind can become free to be an open and focused channel. According to the *Yoga Sutras* we take 21,600 breaths per day. In today's busy world we exceed this level, so our lifespan diminishes. Yoga slows down breathing, therefore increasing longevity and overall vitality.

When you practise yoga you are dedicating some time only to you. The key to this is to stay focused on what is actually happening to your body via your breath. By being aware, you are opening and expanding your body, bringing in lightness and grace and a lack of restriction (see Pranayama p.28).

Prana = Energy/Breath
Yama = Discipline

Air is cultivated by creating space in the organs and joints, especially in the lungs. The arena of air is the thorax, its source the throat, its medium the skin and nerves, and its control the limbs. Creating air requires using movement while the sign of its presence is its opposite: stillness. Yoga is full of opposites.

Creating air through movement is done via vinyasa or ullolas. *Ullola* is the Sanskrit word for "wave", and suggests using the energy of water to synchronize movement and

breath. They are the "transient fluidity between postures" that help to prepare the body for movement, maintain body temperature, soften the internal muscle cells and tissues, and continue the flow of awareness and internalization of action.

There are a number of variable sequences that are designed to counterbalance the preparation for the posture in readiness for the next. There are several varieties of this in the vinyasa section (see p.40).

However ullolas are a useful medium for practising your awareness of your breathing in relation to the movements performed, while preparing your body safely for further opening and softening. Sometimes vinyasas can be performed aggressively, or too fast, this often happens when correct sensitivity of the breath has not been refined first through using ullolas. Ullolas also give us a chance to re-establish the free rhythm of our breathing away from the controlled breathing of pilates movements and the challenge that comes from doing different posture work.

Perform these two simple ullolas, refining your application of the synergetic relationship between the breath (internal dynamic) and the body (external dynamic). Always perform them with honesty and sensitivity.

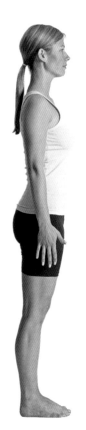

Standing breathing preparation I
Urdvahastullola

This position refines the breath, elongates the spine, broadens the rib cage, and empties the abdomen.

* Stand upright in tadasana (see p.41).
* Distribute your weight across the balls of the feet, widening your foundation. Check for equal pressure across the balls of your feet and heels.
* Gently pull in your thigh muscles, gently engaging your thighs.
* Soften your buttocks, pelvic floor, and your face.
* Inhale through your nose and extend your trunk upwards from the pelvis, comfortably lifting your hips.
* Exhale through your nose and flatten your pubic abdomen towards your spine, stabilizing your lumbar spine.
* Keep your shoulders down, and your neck and head light and long.
* Extend your arms, pointing your fingertips, and keep your eyes, ears, and brain soft.
* Inhale through your nose and raise your arms out and then upwards above your head.
* Look up in-between your palms (do not do this if you have a neck problem).
* Feel the elongation in your spine, your full, broad rib cage, and your empty, hollow abdomen.
* Exhale through your nose, and bring your arms back to your thighs, keeping elongation of the spine, a broad chest, and an empty and hollow abdomen.
* Repeat, lifting arms on inhalation and lowering arms on exhalation, broadening and emptying further with each cycle of breathing.
* Repeat a minimum of 12 times, refining the exact timing of your breathing with your body movement.
  Note: if you have untreated high blood pressure, just bring arms to shoulder height.

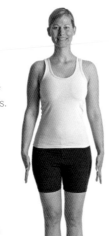

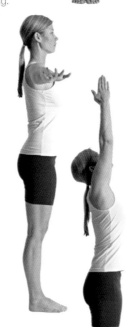

Breathing preparation II
Utkullola

This position develops perfect breathing and body synchronization. It uses the major muscles of the legs and abdomen to heat the body in preparation for vinyasa or asana.

* Stand with your feet together. Balancing across the balls of your feet, widening your foundation. Check for equal pressure across the balls of your feet and heels.
* Keep both legs straight, with the thigh muscles pulled inwards towards the thigh bones, and with the calf muscles lifting the shin bones.
* Soften your buttocks, pelvic floor, and your face.
* Make sure your spine is long, your chest broad, and your abdomen hollow.
* Inhale, push your hips out to bend your knees, and extend both arms long out in front of you.
* Keep the balls of your feet, ankle joints, and inner knees pressed together for stability.
* Continue inhaling until your arms and legs extend back to standing.
* Raise your arms out and then upwards to above your head.
* Look up between your palms (do not do this if you have a neck problem).
* Feel the elongation in your spine, your full, broad rib cage, and your empty, hollow abdomen as before.
* Exhale through your nose, and bring your arms back to your thighs, keeping your spine elongated, a full broad chest, and an empty and hollow abdomen.
* Continue on the next inhalation to push back through the hips, bending the knees, and extend your arms upwards so that you come back up to standing.
* As you exhale, repeat the movement with your arms drawing downwards to your sides and back to the beginning.
* Continue the fluidity of flow between each ullola completing a minimum of 12 cycles.

movements

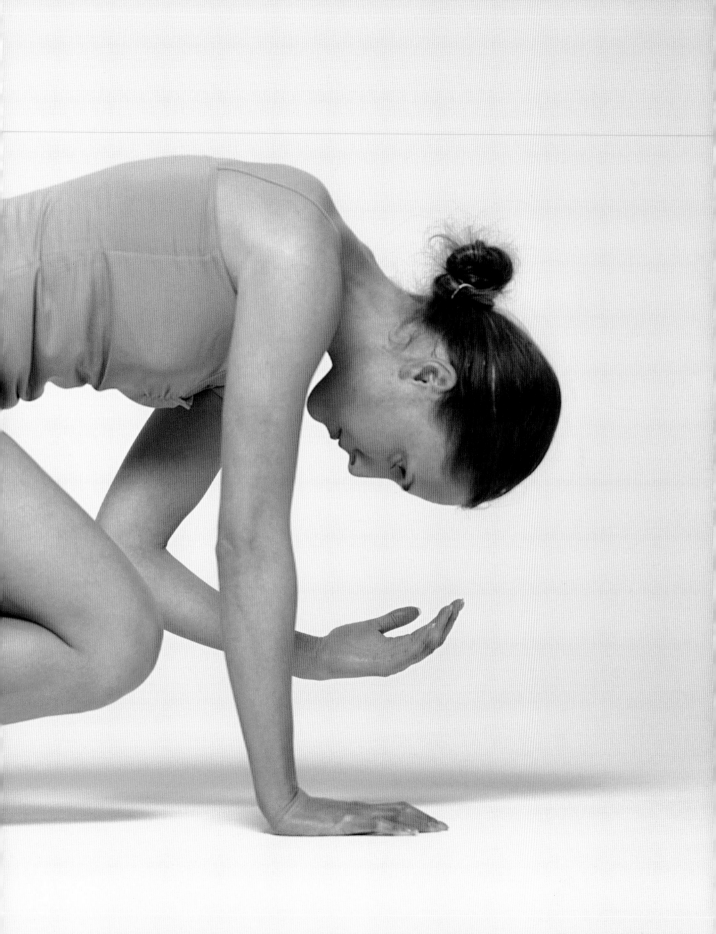

yoga movement preparation

Yoga vinyasa warm-up sequence

This sequence, commonly known as the Sun Salutation, increases understanding of breath and body synchronization following on from the yoga ullolas (see pp.36–7). A vinyasa is primarily used to heat the body in preparation for isolated posture work but it can also be used between your movements to maintain body temperature and aid concentration.

There are two levels of vinyasa, referred to as primary and secondary. It is best to master the primary postures (shown here as easier alternatives) before moving onto the secondary. Follow the instructions given and take each posture on its own before attempting the whole sequence.

Having mastered a vinyasa, it may take anything from 40 seconds to two minutes to complete, depending on your breathing rate. These yoga movements prepare for the softening of the internal connective tissue and muscles, and open the joints.

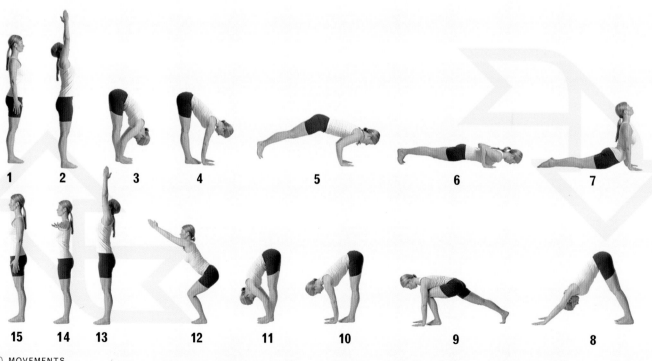

1   2   3   4   5   6   7

15   14   13   12   11   10   9   8

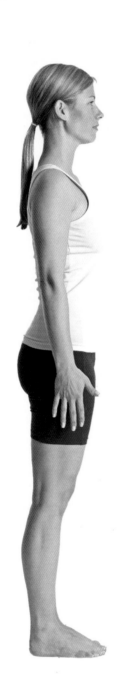

1 ◄ MOUNTAIN POSE
TADASANA

BENEFITS

Gives balance in the body and centres the mind.

* Stand upright with your feet together, keeping them broad and stable. Keep your legs braced and your trunk long.
* Keep your arms long by your side, with your chest open and your shoulders back.
* Hold your jaw straight and parallel to the ground with your face, eyes, and ears soft. Keep your abdomen pulled in, and breathe softly and steadily.

2 ► STANDING, ARMS EXTENDED
URDHVA HASTASANA

BENEFITS

Lengthens the spine, opens the lungs, and improves posture.

* Inhale through your nose and raise your arms out and upwards above your head.
* Look up between your palms (do not do this if you have a neck problem).
* Feel the elongation in your spine, your full broad rib cage, and your empty, hollow abdomen.
* Hold the position while looking at your palms and keeping the core of your body soft. Maintain the charge in your arms and legs until you are ready to release as you exhale.

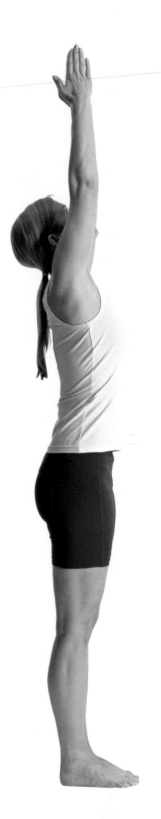

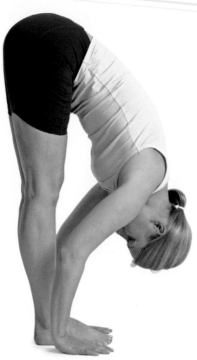

3 ◄ STANDING FOLD
UTTANASANA

BENEFITS

Lengthens hamstrings and hydrates discs between vertebrae.

✳ From a standing position, keep your feet strong and your legs straight, and on your next exhalation pivot your pelvis over your thighs, bringing your chest and head down, placing the palms of your hands on the floor beside your feet.

4 ▼ ACTIVE BACK EXTENSION
ARDHA UTTANASANA

BENEFITS

Opens rib cage and strengthens shoulder retraction and abdominal/spine synergy.

✳ Keeping your armpits lifted away from your hip bones, broaden your rib cage, and suck your solar plexus in and up keeping the chest active, broad, and full. Feel your long, empty, and passive abdomen as your sacrum and perineum are lifted.
✳ Inhale and extend your trunk. Clarify your flat abdomen and full rib cage as you lengthen your spine, and lift and open your chest, placing your fingertips on the floor in front of your feet.
✳ If you can keep your spine long you can put your palms flat on the floor.

▼ EASIER ALTERNATIVE
BENT LEG FOLD

✳ If you have a back condition or tight hamstrings, bend your legs as you do Standing Fold.

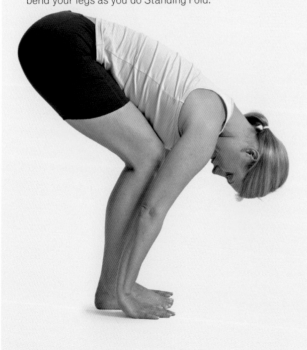

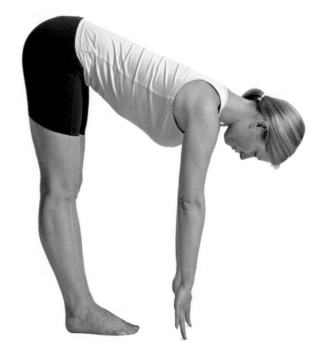

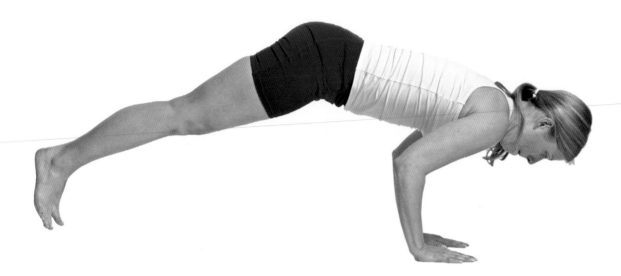

5 ▲ JUMP BACK

BENEFITS

A step action mobilizes the hips, while a jump creates more energy.

❋ Before you do a jump, first practise the easier step-back movement below. When you feel confident with the pose, and have increased your hip mobility and strength, attempt the jump back by inhaling, exhaling, and jumping your legs back. Lift your hips as you jump your legs back and land firmly on the balls of your toes.

TIP

When you jump, take your weight into your hands and push from your arms and shoulders as you lift your body up and take your legs back. You should land with your elbows bent. Do not jump if you are pregnant or if you have a knee injury.

► EASIER ALTERNATIVE STEP BACK

❋ Exhale and press weight evenly into every finger on your hand. Take your weight forward and into your arms as you step your feet back alternately onto the balls of your feet (see above).

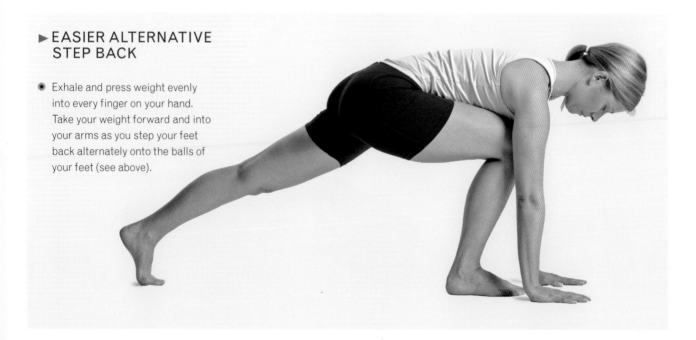

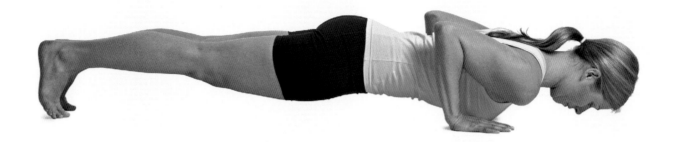

6 ▲ ALL FOURS STAFF POSE
CHATURANGA DANDASANA

BENEFITS

Strengthens chest, arms, and triceps and teaches use of legs and hands in weight-bearing movement.

✳ As you are still exhaling from the jump, bend your elbows right down so that your upper arms are parallel to the floor, your spine is extended, your legs are engaged and strong, and your foundation is your hands and the balls of your toes.

✳ Bring your chin so that it is about an inch from the floor, keeping your chest, pelvis, and knees off the floor. Look down to your nose and the floor.

✳ Press your weight evenly onto the broad balls of both feet, fully engaging your legs by sucking your thigh muscles into your thigh bones.

✳ Make sure your hands have full contact with the floor, keeping your palms broad and fingers long as they press downwards.

▼ EASIER ALTERNATIVE
ARDHA CHATURANGA DANDASANA

✳ Instead of using the hover position of chaturanga dandasana you may find it easier to bend your knees and rest your chest on the floor. This is a half version (*Ardha* in Sanskrit).

✳ It is common not to have the upper-body strength necessary to lower into the All Fours Staff Pose without collapsing the pelvis. Do try to avoid this as it causes lower spinal pain.

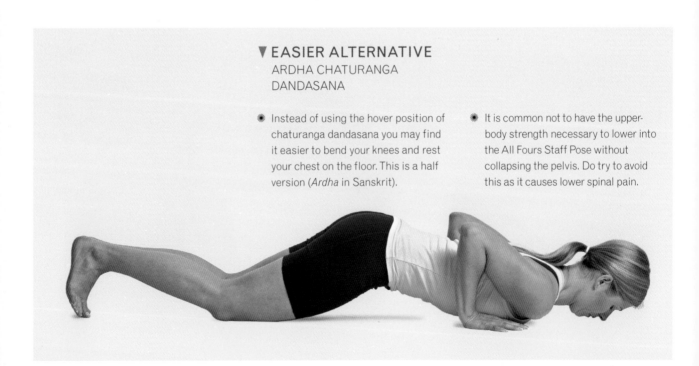

7 ▶ UPWARD FACING DOG
URDHVA MUKHA SVANASANA

BENEFITS

Rejuvenates the spine and strengthens the shoulders and arms.

* As you inhale, push your chest forward, straighten your arms, and push down your toes into Upward Facing Dog position.
* Make sure that your knees and hips are off the floor with this movement.

TIP

Rolling over your toes will happen naturally if you keep your feet where they are and come into Upward Facing Dog by pressing your chest forward and straightening your arms. If you take your hips back initially you should gain enough momentum to press forward through your arms and chest and to roll onto your toes.

▶ EASIER ALTERNATIVE

* Instead of coming into Upward Facing Dog position, inhale and come back onto all fours. It is better to practise this pose first, until your understanding of the breathing technique refines.
* When you are used to this position, you can practise Upward Facing Dog, keeping your knees on the floor, but be careful that your pelvis does not collapse and that you have built up enough upper body strength first, practising the All Fours Staff Pose.

TIP

If you suffer from a back condition, only practise this easier alternative of Upward Facing Dog.

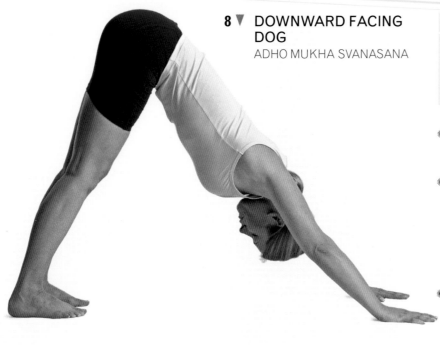

8 ▼ DOWNWARD FACING DOG
ADHO MUKHA SVANASANA

BENEFITS

Aids digestion, lengthens legs and spine, and refines the use of hands and feet.

* As you exhale, push up your buttocks and roll over your toes, pushing them into Downward Facing Dog.
* Relax your head and neck completely, keeping your hands a shoulder-width apart, and keeping your feet parallel and a hip-width apart. Your back is extended, your shoulders are strong, and your arms and legs are straight.
* Focus on Uddiyana bandha (see p.31) and correct breathing by opening the front and back of your rib cage, expanding your rib crests, and hollowing your pubic abdomen (see also p.37).

► EASIER ALTERNATIVE

* If you find the position hard, bend your knees until you feel your body soften and your hamstrings beginning to release. Be patient and the full Downward Facing Dog position will be possible if approached with sensitivity and honesty.

TIP

When you feel your body has softened and is warmer, you can hold this position for a little longer.

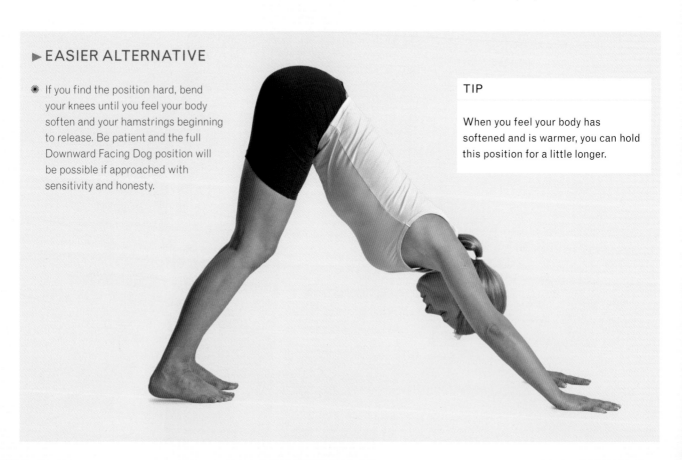

9 ▶ STEP BACK

BENEFITS

Opens the hip joints and strengthens the thighs and trunk.

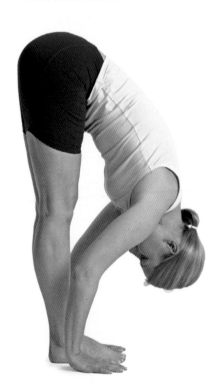

* As you inhale, step your legs forwards alternately with your feet by your hands.
* Soften your knees and press your weight through your hands and arms as you move your back leg forwards, landing softly with both feet in-between your hands.

* Alternatively, jump both feet together in a Jump Back (see p.43). To do this your hands have to be firm on the floor and "grounded."

TIP

Do not use the jumping motion if you cannot ground both hands when in a Standing Fold. The stability through the palms and arms gives you the strength to jump your legs through. Also avoid the jumping movement if you have knee injuries.

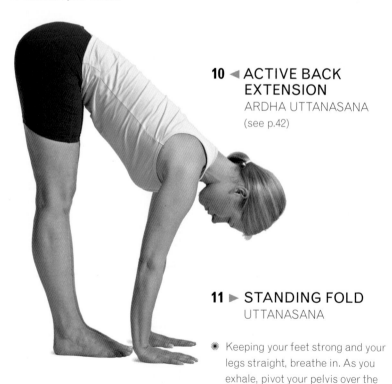

10 ◀ ACTIVE BACK EXTENSION
ARDHA UTTANASANA
(see p.42)

11 ▶ STANDING FOLD
UTTANASANA

* Keeping your feet strong and your legs straight, breathe in. As you exhale, pivot your pelvis over the top of your thighs, placing your palms to the floor on either side of each foot as you go into the fold.

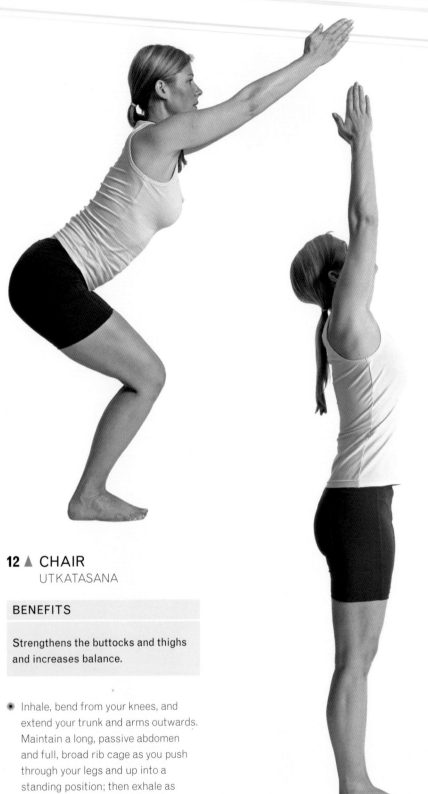

13 ◄ STANDING, ARMS EXTENDED
URDHVA HASTASANA

BENEFITS

Lengthens the spine, opens the lungs, and improves posture.

* Inhale through your nose and raise your arms out and upwards above your head.
* Look up between your palms (do not do this if you have a neck problem).
* Feel the elongation in your spine, your full broad rib cage, and your empty, hollow abdomen.
* Hold the position while looking at your palms and keeping the core of the body soft. Hold the charge in your arms and legs until you are ready to release as you exhale.

12 ▲ CHAIR
UTKATASANA

BENEFITS

Strengthens the buttocks and thighs and increases balance.

* Inhale, bend from your knees, and extend your trunk and arms outwards. Maintain a long, passive abdomen and full, broad rib cage as you push through your legs and up into a standing position; then exhale as your arms come down.

14 ▼ TRANSITION

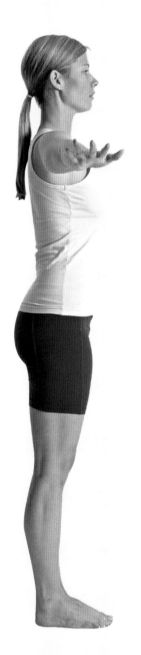

* As you exhale, turn your palms slightly outwards as you release your arms out to the side. Your hands should come down past your shoulders until they are resting next to your thighs with your palms turned inwards.
* Try to time it so that your arms reach your sides at the same time as your final exhalation of breath.

15 ► MOUNTAIN POSE
TADASANA

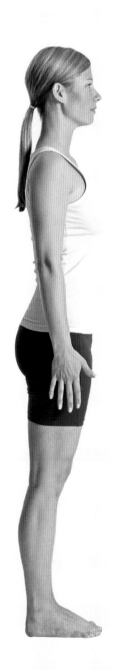

* Stand straight and maintain an empty abdomen and broad rib cage while keeping the core of your body soft. Be aware of any different shifts in sensations as you enjoy the benefits of vinyasa practice.

GUIDELINES

Repeat the warm up sequence 4–12 times, noticing how body heat is produced. This heat is very healing.

TIP

Vinyasas should nourish the body and form gentle movements. Each time you practise try to refine the techniques. Do not be tempted to speed up your breath so that it feels unnatural. The breath will tell you everything; just listen to it and act accordingly.

pilates movement preparation

Pilates-based warm-up sequence

These pilates warm-up exercises have been chosen to teach you correct neutral alignment and breathing in some of the more simple postures before you move on to do the harder movements. Pilates is designed to teach you how to re-align your spine as you tone and lengthen the surrounding muscles. Notice any difference, or any changes you feel as you practise the pilates warm-up and make your own comparisons to the yogic vinyasa (see pp.40–49).

As you practise these pilates techniques pay particular attention to your breathing, especially when you exhale, as in pilates the exertion is always on the exhalation. When you exhale you will either hollow your abdomen inwards or practise the pelvic floor lifts. The step-by-step instructions will tell you when to breathe and engage, and it is attention to these details that make pilates movements so effective at strengthening all the deep core muscles of your trunk.

An important difference to note between pilates and yoga is the engagement of the pelvic floor. In pilates you consciously lift the pelvic floor to strengthen and tone the deep abdominal muscles and the spine. However, in yoga the pelvic floor engages as a reaction to deepening the exhalation – as you hollow in your belly, your pelvic floor engages naturally.

When you do these pilates movement preparations, you will feel more support, especially around your body's core area. Make a special effort to feel the pelvic floor zipping up or engaging as you work through the warm-ups. Look back to pp.24–7 if you need to remind yourself about the key principles.

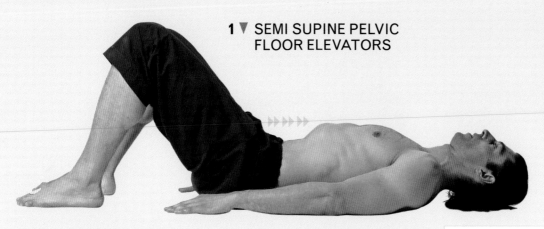

1 ▼ SEMI SUPINE PELVIC FLOOR ELEVATORS

✳ Lie comfortably in the neutral alignment position (see p.32–3)
✳ Check that your pelvis is in neutral spine.
✳ Inhale, broadening your rib cage and lengthening your neck.
✳ Exhale and gently zip your pelvic floor muscles to a 10% hold. Feel your abdominals sink back towards your spine.

✳ Imagine your pelvic floor is like an elevator with three floors. Inhale, then exhale and lift your pelvis gently to the first floor and hold briefly.
✳ Hold this engagement as you breathe in, and as you breathe out zip up your pelvic floor to 20% or the second floor. Inhale and hold briefly.
✳ As you exhale zip up your pelvic floor to 30% or third floor. Inhale and hold briefly before exhaling.

TIP

Achieving a 30% pelvic floor engagement is more effective at strengthening your core than hollowing your abdominals inwards. Get used to this engagement before adding movement.

2 ▼ PELVIC FLOOR LIFT

BENEFITS

This improves body posture and bladder control, flattens the stomach, and may also heighten sexual sensation.

✳ Adopt the spine stretch position shown here. Check that there is a fist width of space between your knees.
✳ Clench your hands as fists and place them on top of each other to make a prop for your spine and head so that they relax.Inhale deeply and fill out your lungs comfortably.
✳ Exhale slowly to a count of six, and lift the muscles between your tailbone and the front of your pelvis as high as you can.
✳ As you finish exhaling, contract your outer muscles that are higher

up in your abdomen. This helps to lift the pelvic floor higher as you squeeze the last air out.
✳ Imagine that your pelvic floor is rising as high as your chest.
✳ Release the movement and then, with a gentle downpush, relax your pelvic floor.
✳ Practise this step four more times, taking a short breath in between each repetition.

TIP

This exercise can restore tone to a pelvic floor weakened by an inactive lifestyle, illness, or childbirth. As the pelvic muscles strengthen they balance various muscles that interact with them. Try this alternative pelvic floor lift, refining your contraction from the previous exercise.

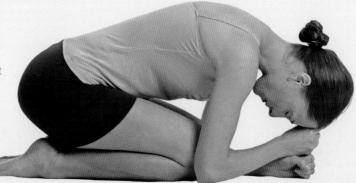

3 ▶ SUPINE ARM RAISES

BENEFITS

Teaches core stabilization and warms up the spine and shoulder joints.

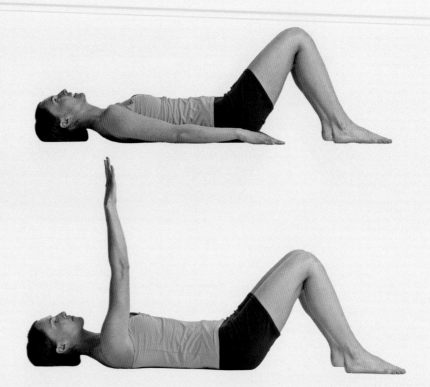

1 Lie in the Relaxation Pose (see p.81) with your legs bent, your feet evenly planted on the ground, and with your spine in neutral position (see pp.32–3).

✻ With your arms down by your side, inhale and fill out your rib cage and broaden your rib crests.

2 Exhale and raise your arms up and over your head, without letting your spine arch away from neutral position.

✻ As you inhale again, release your arms back down to the floor, ensuring your spine does not round into the mat.

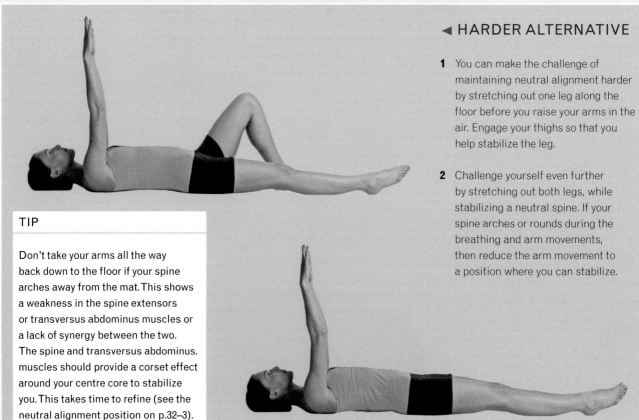

◀ HARDER ALTERNATIVE

1 You can make the challenge of maintaining neutral alignment harder by stretching out one leg along the floor before you raise your arms in the air. Engage your thighs so that you help stabilize the leg.

2 Challenge yourself even further by stretching out both legs, while stabilizing a neutral spine. If your spine arches or rounds during the breathing and arm movements, then reduce the arm movement to a position where you can stabilize.

TIP

Don't take your arms all the way back down to the floor if your spine arches away from the mat. This shows a weakness in the spine extensors or transversus abdominus muscles or a lack of synergy between the two. The spine and transversus abdominus. muscles should provide a corset effect around your centre core to stabilize you. This takes time to refine (see the neutral alignment position on p.32–3).

4 ▶ SPINE ROTATIONS

BENEFITS

Opens the upper body and stretches the chest, while also stabilizing the shoulder blades.

IMPORTANT NOTE

As this exercise involves rotation of the spine, be sure to consult your doctor before attempting it if you have a disc-related injury.

1 Lie on your side with your head on a pillow, knees curled up so that they make a right angle to your body. Keep your back in a straight line, but let it retain its natural curve.

✱ Feel all your bones: shoulders, hips, knees, and ankles resting on top of each other. Extend your arms out in front of you with your palms together at shoulder height.

2 Inhale and and lift your upper arm, keeping your elbow soft and your shoulder blade down. Follow your hand movement with your eyes.

3 Keep following your hand until your arm touches the floor in line with your shoulder.

✱ Keep your knees together and your pelvis stable.

✱ Exhale and bring your right arm, then your left, back to the start position of an arc shape.

✱ Practise the movement five times, then curl up on the other side and repeat.

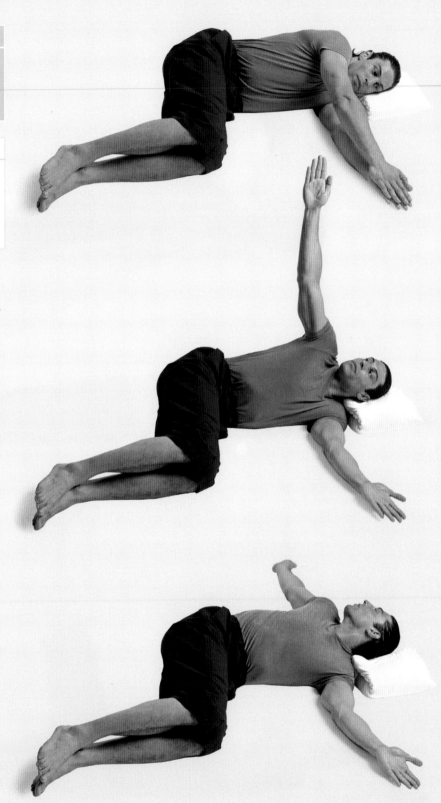

5 ▼ SUPINE LEG RAISES

BENEFITS

Teaches neutral spine position while using heavier leg levers. Tones thighs.

1 Lie in a supine position with both legs stretched out on the floor.
* Ensure that you are in neutral alignment position (see pp.32–3). Pull your right thigh muscle into the thighbone, ensuring that the back of your right knee stays as close to the floor as possible.

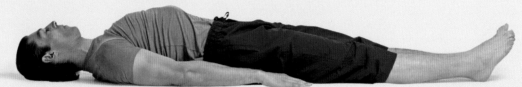

2 Inhale deeply, then exhale, and lift arms up and over your head to rest on the floor.

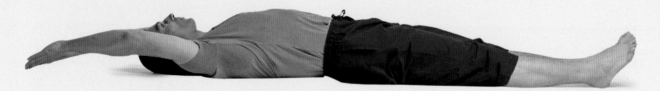

3 Inhale deeply, then exhale, and lift your right leg straight up in the air, without losing the neutral spine; your leg does not have to be perpendicular to your hip.
* Inhale, and hold your leg.
* Exhale, and lower your leg to the floor without resting.
* Practise 10 times, maintaining a neutral spine. Your leg will lift higher as the strength of your abdomen, pelvic floor, and spine improves, then repeat with the other leg.

TIP

You can make the above exercise easier by bending one leg. Suck your left thigh muscles into your thigh bone to engage the leg. Ensure the spine stays in neutral as the heavier lever of the leg is lifted.

6 ▼ THE HUNDRED

1 Lie in the neutral alignment position (see pp.32–3). Engage pelvic stability by hollowing out your pubic abdomen and switching on your pelvic floor muscles.

BENEFITS

Strengthens the abdominal muscles and teaches breath control.

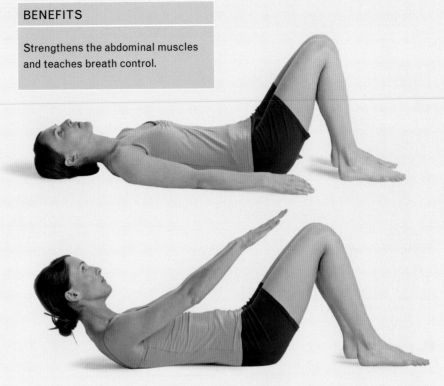

2 Inhale deeply, then exhale, and lift your trunk and arms upwards while maintaining a neutral spine. If your back rounds into the floor do not lift your trunk so high.

* Inhale and exhale again and lift arms quickly into small arm hovers (small rapid movements).

* Inhale for five arm hovers, and exhale for five arm hovers.

* Maintain an elevated trunk but try not to move the trunk – instead stabilize it against your arm hovers. Release back to neutral alignment.

* If five arm hovers are too long for your breath control, then just do four arm hovers per breath until you learn to breathe more efficiently.

* Always breathe through your nose.

▼ HARDER ALTERNATIVE

1 Inhale, and as you exhale zip up your pelvic floor and lift one leg to 90°. Repeat movement as above, keeping a neutral spine.

TIP

To make the movement harder you can try this modification, but work to maintain your neutral spine position. The spine must not arch or slump, but must stay in a neutral, stable position (see pp.32–3).

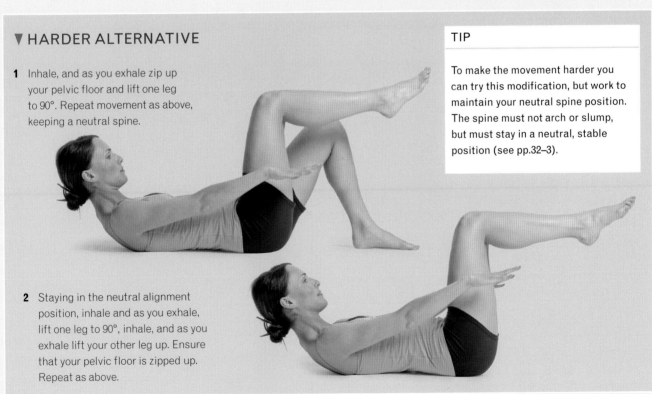

2 Staying in the neutral alignment position, inhale and as you exhale, lift one leg to 90°, inhale, and as you exhale lift your other leg up. Ensure that your pelvic floor is zipped up. Repeat as above.

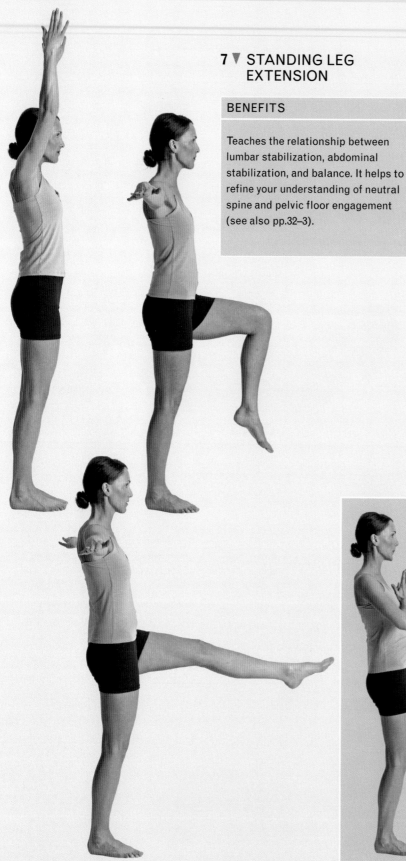

7 ▼ STANDING LEG EXTENSION

BENEFITS

Teaches the relationship between lumbar stabilization, abdominal stabilization, and balance. It helps to refine your understanding of neutral spine and pelvic floor engagement (see also pp.32–3).

1 Stand with your feet together (or hip-width apart if you suffer from a balance problem). Take a neutral stance with your pelvic floor engaged to 20–30 per cent. Keep your shoulders back and relaxed, your face soft, and your neck long.
* Inhale, and as you exhale raise both arms up above your head.

2 Bring your arms down to shoulder height and lift your right knee to a comfortable level. Broaden your rib crests and lengthen your abdomen.

3 Inhale, and as you exhale extend your right leg by flexing your thigh muscle.
* As you inhale take your leg back to the start position with your knee still lifted.
* Practise 8–14 times keeping ears, shoulders, and hips in a straight line; repeat on other side before returning to standing position.

◄ EASIER ALTERNATIVE

* For students who have high blood pressure, or those building strength, release your hands to the prayer position in step 2 as you strengthen your core to stabilize the leg extension.

8 ▼ STANDING SPINE ROLLS

1 Stand with your feet a hip width apart for a stable base. Keep your knees slightly soft and your shoulders back and relaxed. Let your face stay soft and your neck long. Adopt your neutral spine with 20–30 per cent pelvic floor engagement (see p.27).
✳ Inhale to open the front and back lung, and feel your rib cage expanding and your abdomen lengthening.

BENEFITS

These spine curls maintain the health of the inter-vertebral discs that sit in between the bones of your spine. Move with the breath and feel how your spine softens.

2 Exhale and slowly begin to roll your chin towards your chest rolling through every vertebra in your neck, and continue to roll through your upper back.
✳ If you run out of the exhalation, pause. inhale again, and, as you exhale, continue rolling your spine towards the floor like a rag doll.

3 Keep your back rounded but your abdomen must remain actively hollow to protect your spine.
✳ Once you have reached a comfortable level, bend your knees to help your hands to touch the floor, if necessary. Take a few breaths to release your spine, then inhale, and as you exhale draw up your pelvic floor as you roll back your spine to the standing neutral position.

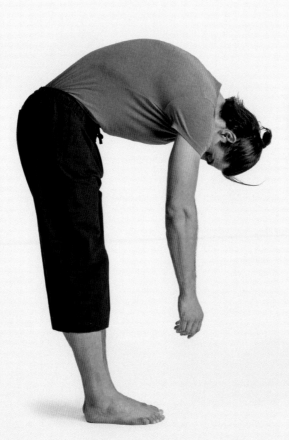
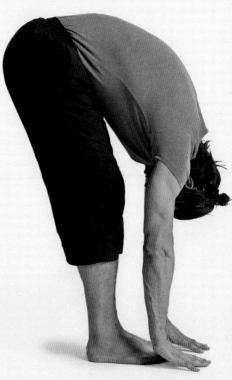

9 ▼ CENTRE PLANK

LEVEL 1 – EASY

1 Kneel in a box position on all fours ensuring that your pubic abdomen is drawn in and up towards your navel, or making sure that the front part of your pelvic floor is engaged.

❋ Rest on your elbows which should be underneath your shoulders, ensuring that your spine stays in a neutral extended position.

HOW TO WORK WITH THE LEVELS

Always work with the correct level for you. You will progress through the levels if you practise as often as you can – ideally 3–5 times a week or 15–20 minutes. Be careful because if you work at the wrong level your body will learn incorrect compensatory movement patterns that are hard to correct.

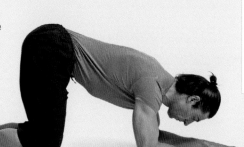

LEVEL 2 – MODERATE

❋ From Level 1 position, inhale and as you exhale pull in your thigh muscles and lift up (engage) your legs so that your knees are off the floor.

❋ Keep your shoulders, hips, and knees in a horizontal line.

❋ On every exhalation refine your abdominal engagement to stop your hips from sinking to the floor and your spine from arching.

❋ Your shoulders should be relaxed and your hands flat.

❋ Hold for 20–60 seconds, then release.

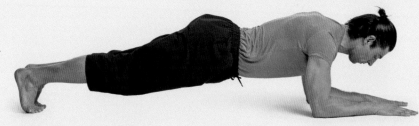

LEVEL 3 – HARD

❋ Once you have built up stabilizing your strength to hold for 40 seconds or more on the moderate plank, try this harder mobile strength plank.

❋ Hold in your moderate plank Level 2, keeping relaxed yet strong. Inhale, and as you exhale lift your right leg off the floor, keeping it long.

❋ Inhale, and bring your right foot back down again.

❋ Exhale, and lift your left leg off the floor, so that your foot lifts right off the floor.

❋ Inhale and take your left foot back down again.

❋ Do not let your hips sink as you lift your leg. Maintain a strong plank position as you start to lift your leg.

❋ Practise 8–14 times before releasing down, keeping a neutral spine and engaged pelvic floor.

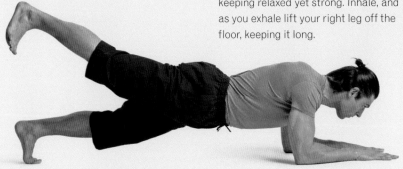

10 ▼ SIDE PLANK

LEVEL 1

✹ Lie on your right-hand side, with your elbow under your shoulder and your legs bent so that they go behind your knees. Keep your knees and hips in line.

✹ Inhale, and as you exhale lift the rib nearest the mat up and away. You can do this by engaging your empty abdomen and the front part of your pelvic floor to make an engagement of 20 per cent.

✹ Keep your shoulders relaxed. Hold for 20–60 seconds.

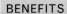

LEVEL 2

✹ Start in the position of Level 1. Inhale, and as you exhale lift your pelvis off the floor. Keep your left hand on your left hip, or try to extend it upwards in line with your shoulder.

✹ Keep refining your pelvic floor engagement.

✹ Look up at your hand for 20 seconds. If you have a neck problem, keep head in line with spine.

LEVEL 3

✹ Start in the position of Level 2. Inhale, and as you exhale extend your left leg out for 20–40 seconds so that it is in line with your hip. More awareness of your neutral alignment will be required to stabilize your pelvis and prevent it from dropping.

✹ Keep your arm up or rest your hand on your hip until you build up strength.

✹ Keep your body in a straight line with parallel hips.

LEVEL 4 – HARDER ALTERNATIVE WITH MOVEMENT

✹ Once you have worked up to holding the previous level for 60 seconds, you can try this harder alternative which includes movement.

✹ Start in the position of Level 3. Inhale, and as you exhale bring your left knee and left elbow towards each other.

✹ Inhale and straighten your leg again, and keep your left arm up in line with your shoulder.
Practise 8–14 times keeping your pelvis stable and your breathing fluid before releasing back down.

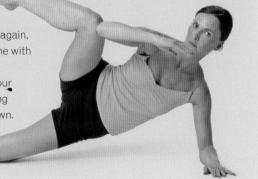

feet, legs, gluteals, and thighs

The standing postures take up the most energy but it is here that you will learn how to use your feet correctly. Learning these positions, using both yoga and pilates poses, transmits strength to the legs and gluteals, building and toning the muscles deeply.

ⓨ CLASSIC WARRIOR SINGLE PLANE
VIRABHADRASANA II

BENEFITS

Opens the pelvis and closes the sacrum.

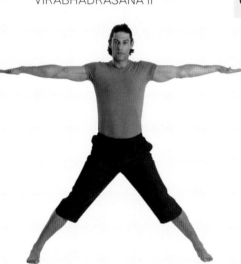 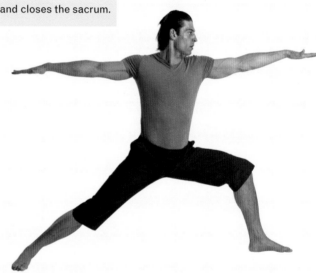

1 Stand upright, inhale, and step your feet out wide – about one and a half shoulder widths apart. Keep your arches lifted and the weight evenly balanced on both feet. Extend your arms to the side, with your biceps rolled slightly back and your forearms rolled slightly forward.

✳ Exhale and extend your little finger out of your rear shoulder, and your index finger out of your armpit.

✳ Inhale and suck your thigh muscles into your bones to protect your knees.

✳ Exhale and brace the outer edges of your feet, opening your pelvis, and feel your outer knees and hips harnessing.

2 Exhale and turn your right foot out 90° and your left foot in 15–25° without allowing your knee to collapse. Keep your heels in line.

✳ Inhale, open your rib cage and fill out your lungs, opening your chest and thoracic spine. Flatten your pubic abdomen to engage the perineum.

✳ Exhale, and engage your leg muscles, moving the outer edge of your left knee backwards. Roll your left hip back, while keeping your right buttock tucked under and your hip stable.

✳ Inhale, and refine your long abdomen and open your full chest.

✳ Exhale, and bend your left leg until it is at a right angle at the knee. Arms stay alive and long.

✳ Look along your left hand. Maintain a strong and long trunk. Keep equal pressure on both feet.

✳ Hold for as long as comfortable refining your technique while maintaining the position.

✳ Inhale and lengthen the spine and abdomen. Exhale and slowly lunge into your left leg.

✳ Inhale, release to the start position. Exhale and repeat.

ʸ CLOSED PLANE EXTENSION
PARSHVOTTANASANA

1 Stand upright, inhale, and step your feet out wide to one and a half shoulder widths apart. Keep weight even.
✳ Exhale maintaining a strong contact of the feet to the floor.

✳ Inhale, and suck your thigh muscles into your bones to protect your knees.
✳ Exhale, brace outer edges of your feet to the floor opening your pelvis. Also feel your outer knees and hips harnessing.
✳ Inhale, and as you exhale take your arms out to the side, parallel to the floor. Your hands are alive, your abdomen is hollow, your chest broad, and your pelvic floor passive.
✳ Breathe rhythmically.

BENEFITS

Lengthens the legs, while releasing lumbar and pelvic tension.

2 Inhale, and as you exhale turn your left foot out to 90° and your right foot in 75° turning the whole leg with it. Line up your heels.
✳ With hands on hips, turn your trunk with your legs to bring left hip forward in line with your right so that your hip bones are parallel.

3 Inhale, broaden your rib crests. Exhale, lengthen your trunk, and extend your spine over your left foot. Keep your pubic abdomen soft and empty.
✳ Retract your shoulders away from the neck and keep your front and back thigh muscles engaged.

✳ Have equal weight on both feet. Feel the opening of your back left calf as you ground your back left foot to bring your left buttock and hip forwards.
✳ Stabilize your right knee in line with your middle toes. Ground the inner and outer edges of your front foot to

TIP

If you feel any discomfort in your knee be sensitive to this limitation and bend your knee slightly.

bring right hip and buttock bone back. Hold briefly then release to standing position, and repeat on other side.

P LUNGE AND BALANCE

BENEFITS

A strengthening movement that incorporates balance while also toning the thighs and reinforcing neutral spine with movement.

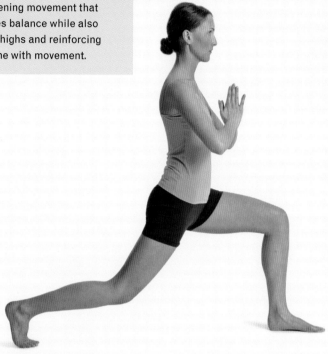

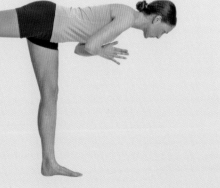

1 Stand upright, then bend your left leg as you step forward and your right leg goes back. Your back right heel will be off the floor.

* Keep equal weight on both feet, pressing your toes into the floor.

* Engage neutral spine with 20–30 per cent pelvic floor engagement. Make sure that your ears, shoulders, and hips stay in a straight line.

* Inhale as you bend both knees to bring your front knee to a 90° angle.

* Keep your pelvic floor engaged and hollow your pubic abdomen towards your spine.

2 Exhale and press your weight through your front foot, drawing your left foot back and inwards towards the back of the right foot.

* Step right foot back to the start position, inhale, and lunge downwards. As you exhale draw your right foot back and inwards again, then repeat on other side.

HARDER ALTERNATIVE

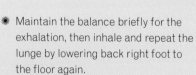

* Inhale, and as you exhale, instead of drawing your back foot inward as in Step 2 try lifting your back right leg by hinging forwards through the hips to counterbalance the leg lift with the trunk lengthening. Do not take your shoulders below hip height.

* Maintain the balance briefly for the exhalation, then inhale and repeat the lunge by lowering back right foot to the floor again.

* Practise 8–12 times, then repeat with other leg.

$\boxed{P}$ $\boxed{Y}$ SHOULDER BRIDGE
SARVANGASANA SETU BANDHA

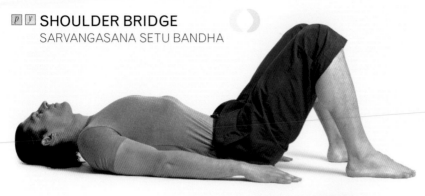

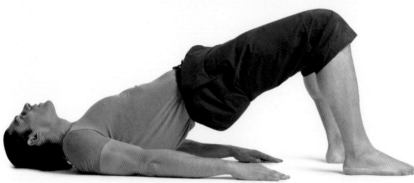

1. Lie on your back with your knees bent, and arms by your side, inhale and as you exhale press your feet evenly into the floor.

   ✳ Inhale, fill out your lungs and chest so that your rib cage becomes broad and active, and allow your abdomen to be long, empty, and passive.

   ✳ Exhale, and press your feet, hands, and shoulders firmly into the floor.

2. Inhale and raise your buttocks and spine slowly off the floor, peeling up each segment of the vertebrae from the sacrum to the top of your spine. Balance on your arms and shoulders and keep your head relaxed.

   ✳ Hold for 5–10 breaths and focus on broadening your rib cage, then inhale, and empty your pubic abdomen as you exhale and slowly roll your spine back down.

HARDER ALTERNATIVE

✳ From Step 1 above, inhale and place your hands each side of your spine as you lift up. Ensure your elbows are directly under your wrists.

✳ Press your shoulders down to facilitate more of a lift.

✳ Hold, breathing evenly for 5–10 breaths, or as long as is comfortable.

✳ Your chin will be tucked into your chest so a very deep nourishing breath will begin to take place. This is *Ujjayi* breathing and will sound like you are breathing with earplugs in. Go with

this natural breath. It still enters and exits through the nose but comes via the throat and palate. It makes a similar sound to when you are clearing your throat.

✳ When you are ready to come down, inhale and as you exhale roll the spine vertebra by vertebra back down to the floor from shoulders to sacrum.

BENEFITS

This posture is a back bend and can aggravate back problems if not performed with care. It tones the front of the body, lengthens the thighs, and opens the chest.

TIP

If you feel that there is too much weight on your neck you are either working on the wrong level or are not pressing through your shoulders enough. If you have a back condition, practise with caution.

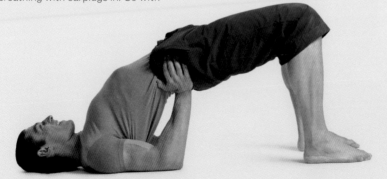

neck, shoulders, arms, and head

If you are suffering from a lack of focus or find it hard to pay attention, it can be due to tension building in the shoulders or arms. This section helps to clear the mind by using movements that help to strengthen upper body muscles and release tension that accumulates around the neck, shoulders, and head.

♪ BIRDIE
BAKASANA

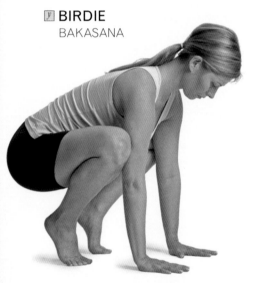

1   Stand with your feet hip-width apart and bend your knees so that you are squatting. Have your arms soft inside your knees and your palms flat on the floor in front of your feet. Inhale.
*   Exhale, and bring your weight forward onto your palms, pressing your outer elbows into your inner knees.
*   Inhale, filling out your chest and emptying your pubic abdomen.
*   Exhale, lifting one foot off the floor, keeping your chest broad. Keep your hands alive, grounding them with your index and little finger.
*   Inhale, keeping equal opposing pressure between the inner knees and outer elbows. Practise with other foot.

BENEFITS

Introduces correct use of your arms and hands while stretching your lower back and groin. It also teaches the relationship of empty and soft core with a full and broad chest to improve balance and strength.

TIP

Practise lifting alternate feet for a while until your strength equalizes – then try to lift both feet.

2   Inhale, and stabilize your head, looking downwards.
*   Lift both feet off the floor at the same time.
*   Exhale, and bring the balls and heels of your feet together.
*   Hold for as long as it is comfortable, releasing down on an exhalation.

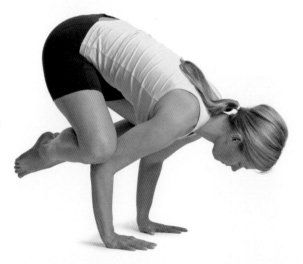

▣ ▣ SPINE EXTENSION
SALABHASANA

BENEFITS

Strengthens the spine and abdomen, while pacifying and slowing the nervous system housed in the central spinal column.

1. Lie flat on the floor with your hands palms down by the sides of your thighs. Place your forehead flat on the floor.
* Keep your shoulders down and away from your ears.
* Inhale, and fill out and broaden your rib cage.
* Exhale, and softly hollow your pubic abdomen inwards towards your spine.

2 Inhale, and exhale to lift your trunk and legs long and away from your centre mid point (you can also lift your trunk and legs separately).
* Holding the position, extend your arms up and away from your trunk.
* Engage your thighs so that your kneecaps are supported and your legs are stable.
* Keep your neck in line with the rest of your spine.
* Feel heat building inside you as you hold the position.
* Hold for as long as comfortable before releasing, breathing freely.

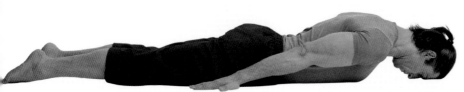

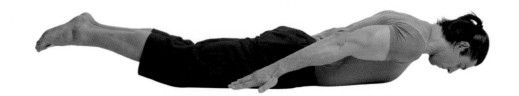

▣ UPWARD FACING BOW POSE
DHANURASANA

1 Lie flat with body and forehead on the floor. Inhale and broaden your rib cage, and as you exhale extend your right arm behind you to grasp your right ankle. Inhale and as you exhale grasp your left ankle with your left hand.
* Breathing evenly, let your pubic abdomen hollow and your chest expand.

2 Inhale, and as you exhale lift your trunk and legs towards each other.
* Extend your trunk out of your pelvis and allow your knees to separate slightly.
* Be aware of balancing on your pelvis as your spine opens. Breathe naturally.
* Inhale, and as you exhale, release back down to a lying position.

BENEFITS

Makes the spine more supple, tones the abdominals, and opens the chest.

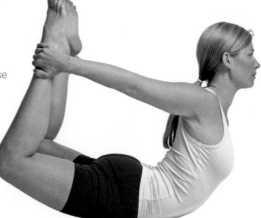

℗ THE SIDE BEND

BENEFITS

Strengthens the waist and shoulders with a laterally positioned core.

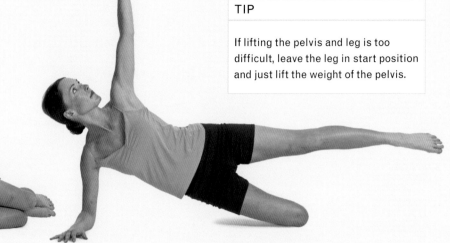

TIP

If lifting the pelvis and leg is too difficult, leave the leg in start position and just lift the weight of the pelvis.

1 Lie propped on your right-hand side on your right arm, with your elbow under your shoulder and your legs bent at the knees, so that your feet are in line with your hips, behind your knees.

2 Inhale, and as you exhale lift up your rib nearest the mat. Extend your pelvis and top leg up and away, engaging your empty abdomen and the front part of your pelvic floor to 20 per cent.
* Keep your shoulders relaxed.
* Inhale, and release your rib, and lift pelvis and leg back to the start position.

* Exhale, and lift your ribs, pelvis, and leg away from the floor, extending your left arm up and over the head into the side bend.
* Keep both hips parallel to each other.
* Inhale, release your rib and arm back down and exhale. Repeat movement on the lift, then repeat on other side.

℗ THE SIDE KICK, KNEELING

1 Start in the same start position as for the Side Bend.
* Inhale, and as you exhale lift up your floating rib nearest the mat. Extend your pelvis and top leg up and away, by engaging your empty abdomen and the front part of your pelvic floor to 20 per cent.
* Keep your shoulders relaxed.
* Extend your left arm high out of the armpit and take your left hand behind your head.

BENEFITS

Tones the thighs and abdomen while strengthening the spine.

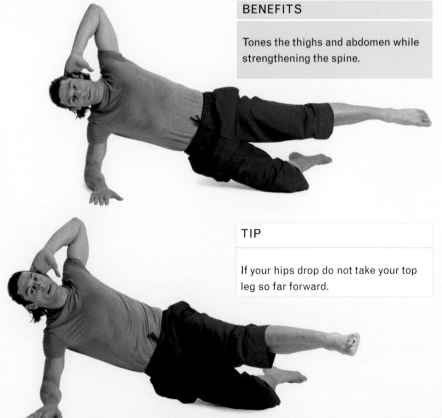

2 Inhale, fill out your rib cage, and as you exhale, extend your left leg forwards maintaining a stable pelvis.
* Inhale, and bring your leg back to the start position.
* Exhale and extend your leg forward, breathing rapidly. Repeat on other side.
* Repeat 8–14 times.

TIP

If your hips drop do not take your top leg so far forward.

₽ THE SPINE STRETCH

BENEFITS

A gentle elongation of the spine to ease tension and rigidity.

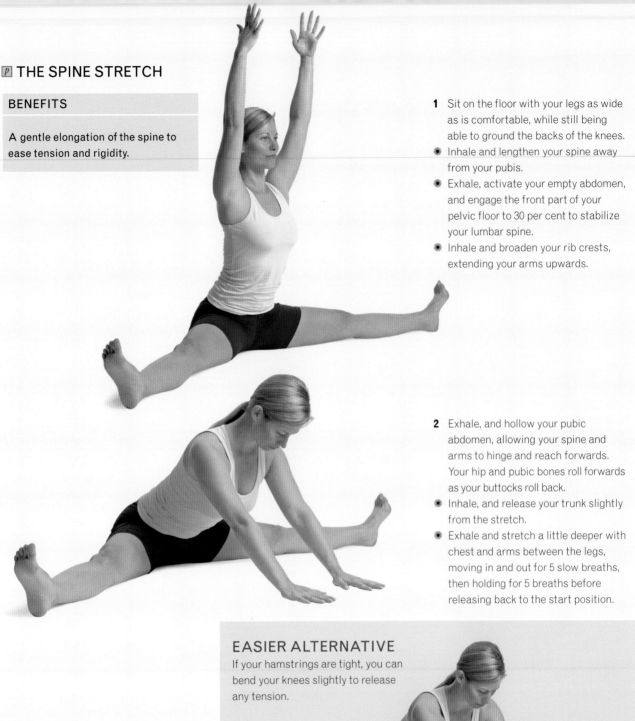

1 Sit on the floor with your legs as wide as is comfortable, while still being able to ground the backs of the knees.
* Inhale and lengthen your spine away from your pubis.
* Exhale, activate your empty abdomen, and engage the front part of your pelvic floor to 30 per cent to stabilize your lumbar spine.
* Inhale and broaden your rib crests, extending your arms upwards.

2 Exhale, and hollow your pubic abdomen, allowing your spine and arms to hinge and reach forwards. Your hip and pubic bones roll forwards as your buttocks roll back.
* Inhale, and release your trunk slightly from the stretch.
* Exhale and stretch a little deeper with chest and arms between the legs, moving in and out for 5 slow breaths, then holding for 5 breaths before releasing back to the start position.

EASIER ALTERNATIVE

If your hamstrings are tight, you can bend your knees slightly to release any tension.

TIP

To really benefit from the stretch, move in and out for 5 breaths, and hold the final position for 5 breaths.

core strength
and abdominals

The core is the most important section of the body for maintaining a healthy spine, as this is the area that gives the whole body its solidity and basic structure. Learning to use the correct muscles around the spine in this section will help to strengthen your abdomen and your whole spinal area.

𝑝 𝑦 BOAT POSE, SUPPORTED
NAVASANA

BENEFITS

Teaches synergy of the abdominals and spine extensors to support the trunk, while strengthening the core.

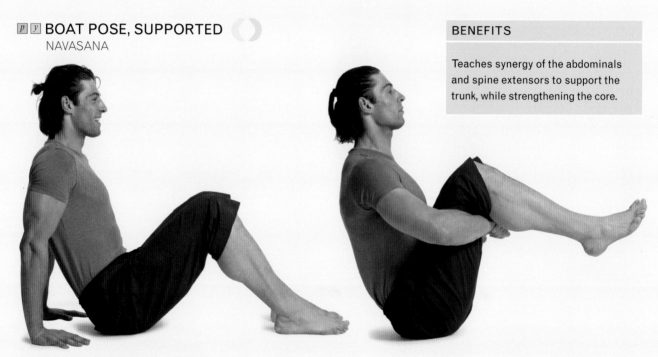

1 Sit on the floor with your knees bent, balancing centrally on the bones of your buttocks with your arms behind you, palms facing forward.

* Inhale and broaden your rib crests. As you exhale, hollow your pubic abdomen towards your spine.

* Clasp your right hand onto your left wrist underneath your thighs.

* Inhale, opening rib cage, then exhale flattening your pubic abdomen and extending your spine.

2 Inhale, and as you exhale start to lift both feet slowly off the floor.

* Stabilize your position by keeping a broad rib cage and a passive and empty abdomen.

* Inhale, stabilize, and as you exhale try to extend your legs away from your trunk, while keeping your back long.

* Hold for as long as comfortable. Inhale, and as you exhale slowly take your legs back to the start position with a controlled movement.

P Y TOE BALANCING POSE

UTTHITA HASTA
PADANGUSTHASANA

BENEFITS

Develops your balance, while strengthening your abdomen and toning your legs.

* Sit on the floor with your knees bent and your arms behind you, palms facing forward. Inhale, and roll back slightly so that you are balancing on your buttocks. Lift your feet off the ground by holding your first two fingers and thumb around the top of your big toes.
* Exhale, and take your feet away from your trunk so that your legs straighten as much as possible.
* Inhale, elevate, and broaden your rib crests, sucking your solar plexus in and up so that your chest becomes active, full, and broad. Your abdomen becomes long, passive, and empty. Engage your flat pubic abdomen as your perineum and sacrum lift in and up.
* Exhale, and hold the position for 3–5 breaths with your legs strong and feet alive, spine long, and waist small before releasing back down towards the floor.
* Keep breathing evenly throughout.

TIP

When practising the harder version, take your legs upwards slowly and hold where you can.

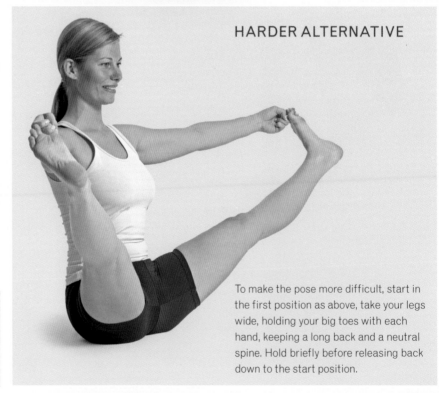

HARDER ALTERNATIVE

To make the pose more difficult, start in the first position as above, take your legs wide, holding your big toes with each hand, keeping a long back and a neutral spine. Hold briefly before releasing back down to the start position.

ⓨ SAGE'S POSE
MARICHYASANA

BENEFITS

This posture works deep into the hip socket, pelvic ligaments, and lower back, while strengthening the core. It releases neck tension and also strengthens the wrists.

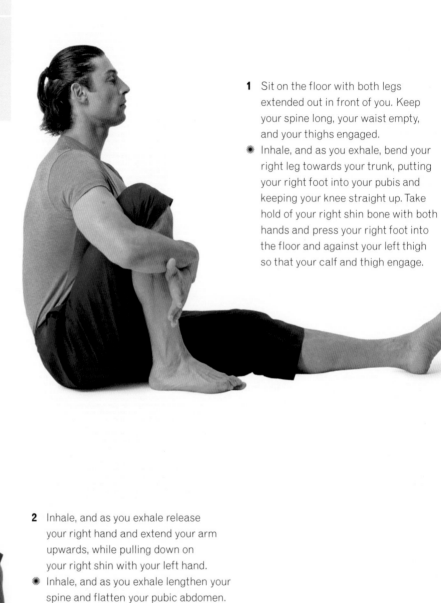

1 Sit on the floor with both legs extended out in front of you. Keep your spine long, your waist empty, and your thighs engaged.

✳ Inhale, and as you exhale, bend your right leg towards your trunk, putting your right foot into your pubis and keeping your knee straight up. Take hold of your right shin bone with both hands and press your right foot into the floor and against your left thigh so that your calf and thigh engage.

2 Inhale, and as you exhale release your right hand and extend your arm upwards, while pulling down on your right shin with your left hand.

✳ Inhale, and as you exhale lengthen your spine and flatten your pubic abdomen.

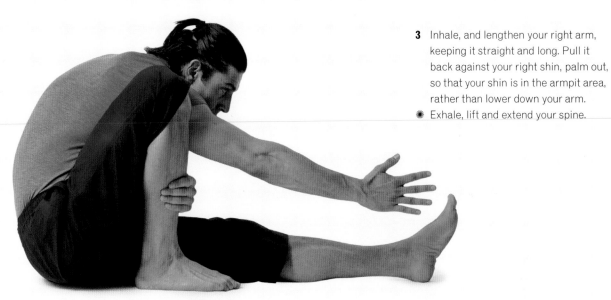

3 Inhale, and lengthen your right arm, keeping it straight and long. Pull it back against your right shin, palm out, so that your shin is in the armpit area, rather than lower down your arm.

✳ Exhale, lift and extend your spine.

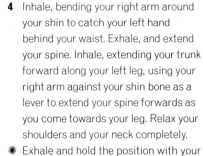

4 Inhale, bending your right arm around your shin to catch your left hand behind your waist. Exhale, and extend your spine. Inhale, extending your trunk forward along your left leg, using your right arm against your shin bone as a lever to extend your spine forwards as you come towards your leg. Relax your shoulders and your neck completely.

✳ Exhale and hold the position with your left thigh muscle engaged and your core soft. Inhale and exhale to release back down when you are ready. Repeat on the other side.

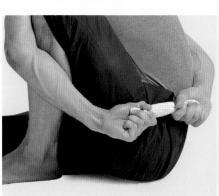

EASIER MODIFICATION

If you can't quite grip behind your back, use a small hand towel and progressively shorten the grip to deeply soften your back muscles.

TIP

If the full movement is too difficult for you, then stay hugging your front shin bone and lengthen your spine away from your sacrum with your breathing.

ⓟ THE ROLL

Strengthens your abdominals and spine against the effects of gravity and momentum.

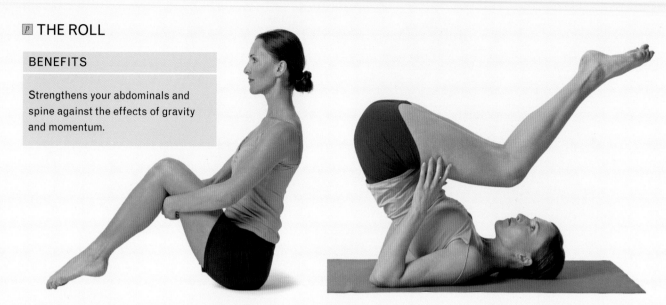

1 Sit with your buttocks on the floor, legs bent. Keep a long spine and abdomen.
* Placing your hands on your shin bones under your knees, gently lift your trunk up and out of your pelvis by activating your abdominals and drawing them in towards your spine.

2 Inhale, and open your rib crests to allow your front and back lungs to fill. Rock back onto your spine, not onto your neck, and press your arms onto the floor as your legs go over your head. Try to keep an equal spacing between your fingers, knees, and chest.

* Exhale, and lift your trunk, rolling back down to the start position with a long spine and abdomen. Try not to dome the abdominals, instead keep them taut to stabilize the spine. Keep fingers evenly spaced with the knees.
* Repeat 8–12 times, breathing evenly.

ⓟ SPINE ROLL DOWNS

BENEFITS

Releases tension in the spine and opens intervertebral discs, while toning your abdomen.

1 Lie flat in the Relaxation Pose (see p.81). Inhale, then exhale and zip up and engage your transversus abdominis into your pubic abdomen.
* Inhale, and as you exhale lift your right leg straight up. Repeat with your left leg, so that both legs are in the air.

2 Inhale, and as you exhale start to roll your legs back, bringing your knees towards your nose and pressing your arms onto the floor.
* Inhale to turn your legs so that they are parallel, and open them a shoulder-width apart.
* Breathe out, keep your abdomen hollow and slowly roll one vertebra at a time back down to the start position.
* Repeat 4–12 times.

TIP

Avoid this movement if you have any neck or back tension.

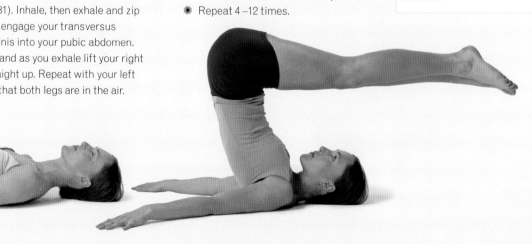

ⓟ DIAMOND PRESS PROGRESSION

BENEFITS

This exercise mobilizes your shoulders while toning your core.

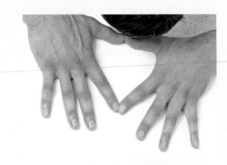

1 Start in the same lying start position as the Spine Extension (see p.65).
* Place your hands in a diamond shape in front of your face with your elbows comfortably wide.
* Inhale, and lift your trunk centre.

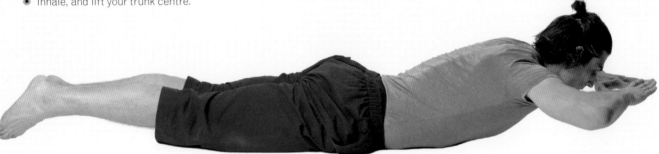

TIP

To make this movement harder, lift your lower legs away from your pelvis at the same time as you lift your trunk.

2 Exhale, and release your arms forward then to your side to bring your hands, with palms up, close to your thighs.
* Inhale, bring your arms out to the side and forward into the diamond shape.
* Exhale, and release the diamond and trunk towards the floor without resting completely.

* Ensure that the balls of your feet remain open and together; your heels can be slightly apart.
* Keep your sacrum open and your buttocks soft.
* Repeat 10–12 times, breathing evenly.

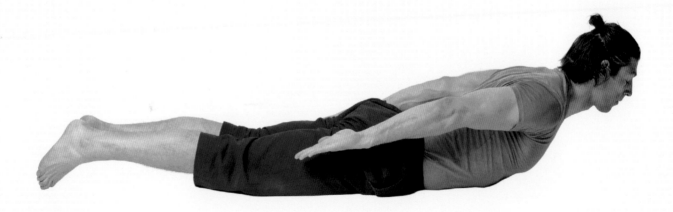

closing postures

These closing postures are excellent for releasing deep spinal tension. A certain strength needs to be gained from the previous section to complete some of the more challenging movements. It is very important to take your time and work at the correct level for you. Students who have a history of serious back trouble or are pregnant should avoid these movements and go straight to the counter poses and relaxation section.

♪ HALF FOETUS, SUPPORTED

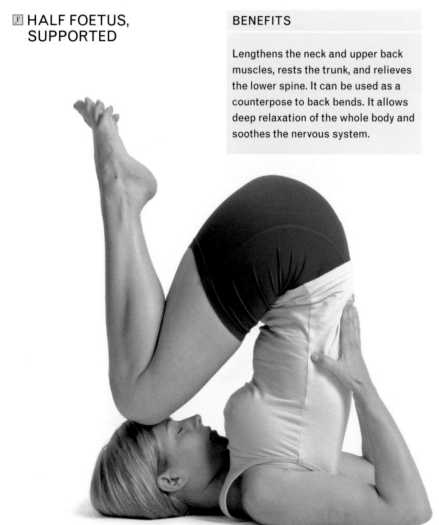

BENEFITS

Lengthens the neck and upper back muscles, rests the trunk, and relieves the lower spine. It can be used as a counterpose to back bends. It allows deep relaxation of the whole body and soothes the nervous system.

1 Lie flat on the floor with your legs bent and your feet flat on the floor.

* Keep your shoulders, arms, and palms flat on the floor.

* Inhale, and push your lower body upwards over your trunk and bring your knees towards your forehead.

* Exhale, and hollow and empty your abdomen.

* Inhale, and bring both hands underneath your pelvis to support your spine with your palms facing upwards.

* Keep your elbows in line with your wrists.

* Press your shoulders back into the floor with your legs bent and your heels by your buttocks.

* Breathe evenly and naturally.

* Hold for as long as is comfortable.

* Inhale, place your hands back onto the floor, and as you exhale slowly roll your spine back down vertebra by vertebra as you release your breath.

▣ FOETUS POSE
KARNAPIDASANA

BENEFITS

A deeply internalizing posture that opens the spine and focuses your breath release.

1 Start in the Half Foetus. Inhale, and as you exhale release your arms behind you to use the floor for support.
✳ You can stay here for a short while and get used to the breathing and internalization.
✳ Release your knees from your forehead so that they release onto the floor above your head.

2 Inhale and as you exhale extend your arms along your ears one arm at a time. Bring your knees over your forehead by your ears while clasping your opposite shins.
✳ Maintain an empty, hollow, and passive core and a full broad rib cage. Keep your pelvic floor passive until your hollow pubic abdomen initiates the pelvic floor to lift up and in.
✳ Hold until your breath is soft and slow; then release back down.

> **TIP**
>
> If you feel any pressure in your neck you need to use your shoulders more, keeping them open rather than collapsing them in towards the chest.

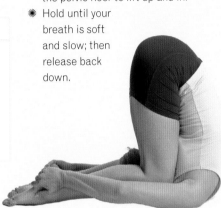

▣ FULL PLOUGH
HALASANA

BENEFITS

This posture is the most nourishing yoga posture as it pacifies the nervous system, lengthens the spine, and rests all the internal systems.

1 Start in Foetus Pose. Inhale, and as you exhale slowly lengthen your legs away from your forehead keeping your arms supporting your spine.

> **TIP**
>
> You could pile up some cushions or a folded blanket and rest your feet on them until your spine lengthens and your breathing refines.
>
> Do not perform this pose if you have a neck problem, just stay in the Half Foetus position.

2 Inhale, and as you exhale straighten your legs by engaging your thigh muscles.
✳ Keep the balls of your feet broad and your abdomen empty.
✳ Keep pressing your shoulders into the floor with your neck relaxed.
✳ Release your arms one by one to the floor as this posture can be maintained without arm support.
✳ Check that you can ground both balls of your feet to support the spine. If you cannot ground your feet, stay in Foetus Pose until your spine and hips have released and softened.

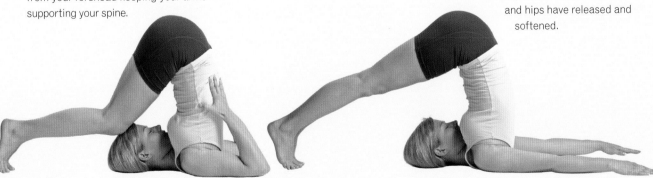

⅄ HALF SHOULDER STAND PREPARATION

BENEFITS

This preparation for Half Shoulder Stand strengthens the wrists and upper trunk and teaches pivotal movement of the pelvis. Check that you are pivoting from the pelvis and not just raising your legs.

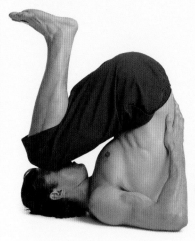
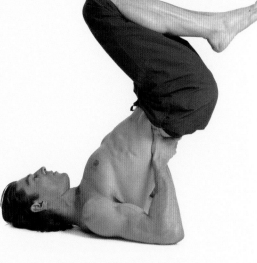

1 From the Half Foetus pose (see p.74) place your hands underneath the back of your pelvis with your feet evenly held in the air.
* Balance your knees on or near your forehead, and keep your shoulders pushed down into the floor.

2 Inhale. and as you exhale gently rock your pelvis back into your hands.
* Inhale and bring your knees back down to your forehead
* Exhale and pivot your pelvis through your hands so that it drops back into your hands with your knees bent.
* Practise moving your pelvis forwards and back without lifting your legs before releasing down.

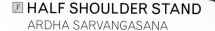

⅄ HALF SHOULDER STAND
ARDHA SARVANGASANA

BENEFITS

Strengthens shoulder and arms as you lift trunk upwards.

* Start in the Half Foetus pose (see p.74). Inhale, and as you exhale take your pelvis back into your hands.
* Inhale and broaden your rib crests. As you exhale, engage your thigh muscles and extend your legs away from your pelvis – your feet are over your head and your pelvis behind your trunk.
* Inhale, and as you exhale broaden though the balls of your feet.
* Keep breathing evenly with your legs strong and feet alive.
* Hold for as long as comfortable keeping your pelvis supported by your hands.
* Inhale, as you exhale bring your knees back to your forehead and your heels towards your buttocks.
* Inhale as you release your arm foundation back to the floor.
* Exhale and roll down through your spine releasing the back and resting in any of the counter poses on pp.80–81.

⚅ SHOULDER STAND
SALAMBA SARVANGASANA

1 Start in Half Foetus pose (see p.74). Inhale and as you exhale lift your trunk up higher by bringing your open palms higher up your spine towards the ribs.
* Inhale, and as you exhale straighten your legs upwards, engaging your thigh muscles.
* Keep your feet broad with your legs together.
* Press through your shoulders to gain more lift in your trunk and lift your hips away from the supported position.
* Keep your feet, knees, hips, and shoulders in a straight line. Maintain the lift with your full and broad rib cage and empty passive abdomen.
* Hold for as long as comfortable.

TIP

You can counterbalance these inversions with the sequence of movements that are detailed in the next section.

BENEFITS

Another deeply nourishing yoga posture that increases blood supply to your face and brain while strengthening your upper body.

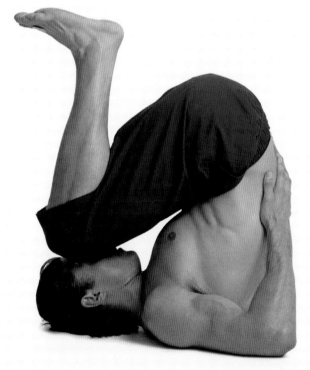

2 Inhale, and as you exhale bring your knees back down to your forehead.
* Inhale and release your arms back down to the floor.
* Exhale and roll your spine down to the mat, verterbra by verterbra, from your thoracic spine to your sacrum.
* Reground yourself as you exhale fully.

HEADSTAND
SIRSASANA

DOLPHIN PRESS
START POSITION

* Starting on all fours on the floor, clasp your fingers together and place them on the floor so that your shoulders and elbows are level and in line.
* To find the area on your head that you will use as a foundation, place your fingers in your ears and trace a line to the centre of your head. This should be just before the crown.
* Assume a Downward Facing Dog position (see p.46).
* Inhale, and as you exhale press through your shoulders as you place your head on the floor cradled by your hand grip.
* Practise taking weight away from your head first. When you feel stronger, walk your feet in a little closer. Be careful not to roll over your head.
* Take frequent rests in Child's Pose (see p.81).

TIP

It is recommended that you stay at these basic levels for weeks or months, improving your trunk, shoulder, and abdominal strength before trying the full Headstand.

TIP

70 per cent of your weight should be absorbed by your shoulders and trunk, and 30 per cent by your head.

BENEFITS

An internalizing posture that aids circulation and increases blood supply to the face and brain. To get safely into a Headstand requires a significant amount of abdominal strength which is why you should follow the steps outlined before trying the full posture.

DOLPHIN
ONE LEG LIFT HEADSTAND PREPARATION

* From the start position, inhale, and as you exhale lift upwards through your trunk, shoulders, and abdomen and balance on the tips of your toes.
* Hold for as long as comfortable, and then rest.

DOLPHIN
TOE TIP HEADSTAND PREPARATION

* From Toe Tip Headstand preparation, inhale, and as you exhale try lifting one foot off the floor.
* Alternate legs a few times before coming down to rest.

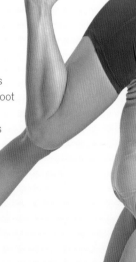

HALFWAY HOUSE
TWO LEG LIFT

❋ From Toe Tip Headstand preparation, inhale, and as you exhale slowly lift both feet together and hold them halfway up.
❋ Use your shoulders, trunk, and abdomen to maintain this position.
❋ Inhale, and as you exhale slowly come down with both feet together.

TIP

If you have to kick up to get into your Headstand you will damage your neck. This is a sign that your abdomen is weak and momentum is required to lift your legs. Do not continue with this method, but practice against a wall, gradually walking your legs up the wall into Two Leg Lift.

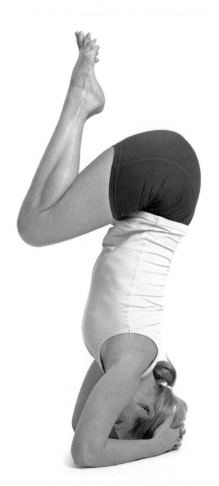

ONE LEG EXTENSION HEADSTAND

❋ From the Two Leg Lift position, inhale and as you exhale extend one leg. Hold briefly, then release down.
❋ Inhale, and as you exhale repeat from the start, extending the other leg.

TIP

The more practice you have doing this posture the smoother your technique will become.

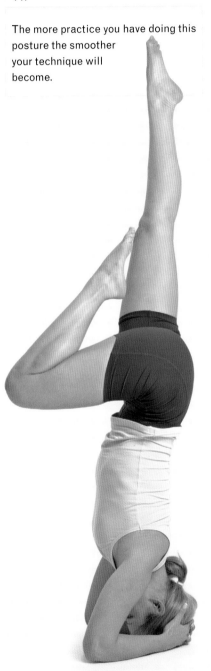

FULL HEADSTAND

❋ After you have practised One Leg Extension, inhale, and as you exhale extend both legs upwards.
❋ Keep your trunk strong and shoulders alive, your abdomen hollow, and rib cage broad using the bandhas (see p.31). Hold, then come down slowly, resting in the Two Leg Lift position before curling back down.

TIP

After inversions, always make sure you rest for at least 10–15 minutes in the yoga Relaxation Pose (see p.81). These steps will take you a while to work through but they ensure that you learn the technique correctly. So many books fail to teach the vinyasa krama (progressions) to this posture.

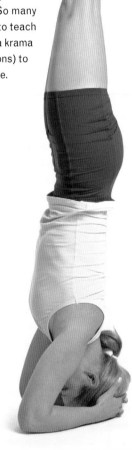

counter poses and relaxation

After your session it is important to use these counterposes to release any tension held in the body, and to rest before getting up. This allows your central nervous system time to rest. Yoga can amplify dormant emotions, so be aware of this. By using this section after practise you deeply nourish your body and prevent the onset of fatigue.

ⓨ SEATED HALF FISH
ARDHA MATSYASANA

1 Sit on your buttock bones with your legs extended out in front of you.
* Inhale, and broaden your rib crests and fill out your lungs.
* Exhale, and make a hollow, soft, and empty abdomen, flattening it towards your spine.
* Take your hands behind your pelvis and inhale, opening your rib cage, with your elbows grounded behind your wrists.
* Exhale and empty your lower abdomen.

EASIER ALTERNATIVE
If the extended legs are not comfortable try this crossed-leg version. Ensure to take your head back from the base of the skull.

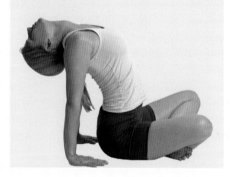

TIP

If you have a neck condition or do not have the upper trunk and arm strength to allow your neck to surrender, do not take the head back. On the inhalation focus on opening your chest, and on the exhalation extend back through your shoulders.

2 Inhale, and extend your head forward from the base of your skull, then upwards and back as you exhale.
* Lift up through your shoulders to surrender your neck to the strength of your arms and trunk.
* Keep your legs active, feet responsive, and your thighs engaged.
* Hold for as long as is comfortable.
* Inhale, and as you exhale lift your head from the base of the skull, upwards, forwards, then down, before releasing back down.

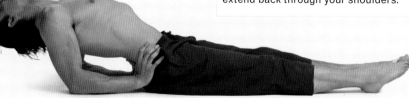

𝒴 CHILD'S POSE
BALASANA

1 Start on all fours. Inhale and fill out your lungs.

✳ Exhale and gently press your buttocks down towards your heels.

✳ With your abdomen hollow, bring two fists underneath your forehead to prop up your spine.

TIP

If your spine feels uncomfortable in this position, place your hands flat under your forehead once your spine lengthens. Placing your hands behind you opens your shoulders and back.

BENEFITS

A spine releasing move that dissipates tension in the tiny intervertebral discs of your spine.

2 To make the pose more passive, you can extend your arms back alongside your feet, with palms facing up, and then relax completely.

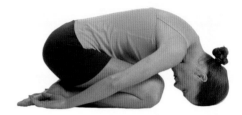

𝓅 𝒴 BUTTERFLY POSE
SUPTA BADDHA KONASANA

BENEFITS

Releases pelvic and lumbar spine tension. Quietens the mind and promotes internalization.

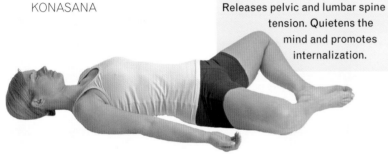

✳ Lie flat on the floor with your legs bent.

✳ Inhale, and put your hands by your side.

✳ Exhale, and allow your knees to drop gently apart and your pelvis to open.

✳ Inhale, and fill out your rib crests. Exhale, and flatten your pubic abdomen.

✳ Allow your breathing to slow down and hold for as long as is comfortable.

𝒴 RELAXATION
SAVASANA

BENEFITS

A deep relaxation pose that offsets any fatigue after yoga practice.

✳ Lie flat on the floor with your legs and arms completely relaxed.

✳ Place your palms face up with your arms about a foot from your body.

✳ Gently lengthen the back of your neck and throat, relaxing your lower spine.

✳ Recognize and then release any residual tension as you exhale softly.

✳ Become aware of the surface of your body and its weight on the floor.

✳ Draw your senses inwards until you feel light, open, and soft.

✳ Feel your whole body deepening as it softens. Feel the tiny connective tissue between your muscles and ligaments melting.

✳ Relax the muscles of your jaw, then your lower spine, softening your pelvic floor and abdomen.

✳ Allow your sensitivity to flow throughout your whole body.

✳ Deeply rest for at least 10–15 minutes.

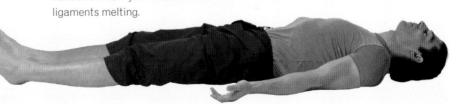

15-minute "busy day" session

This session has been devised for you to incorporate some of the pilates and yoga movements in a short 15-minute work out. One of the biggest excuses for not doing exercise is "lack of time", but this simple routine is quick and therefore easy to fit into your schedule. The session is best done before or after work and should be practised at least three times a week. Try to keep the session flexible, because once you start you may decide that you want to do more or less!

NOTE FOR THE 15-MINUTE AND 30-MINUTE SESSIONS
For each movement there is a page reference which directs you to the step-by-step instructions on how to perform it. Once you are confident that you have mastered each movement and can perform it safely then you will be able to complete the session using the guidelines that follow only.

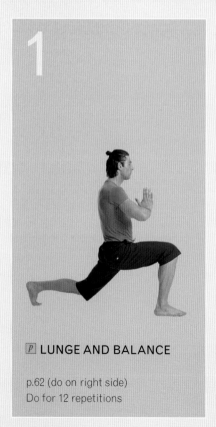

1

ⓟ LUNGE AND BALANCE

p.62 (do on right side)
Do for 12 repetitions

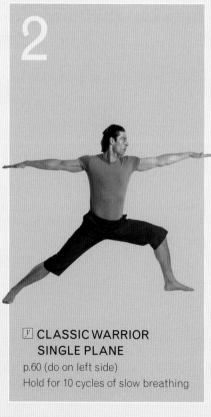

2

ⓨ CLASSIC WARRIOR SINGLE PLANE

p.60 (do on left side)
Hold for 10 cycles of slow breathing

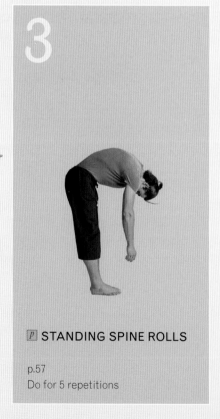

3

ⓟ STANDING SPINE ROLLS

p.57
Do for 5 repetitions

4

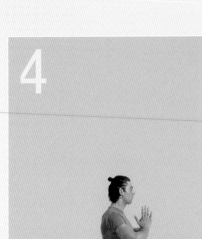

ⓟ LUNGE AND BALANCE

p.62 (do on left side)
Do for 12 repetitions

5

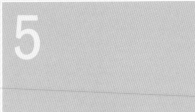
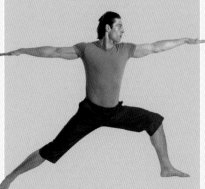

ⓨ CLASSIC WARRIOR
SINGLE PLANE

p.60 (do on right side)
Hold for 10 cycles of slow breathing

6

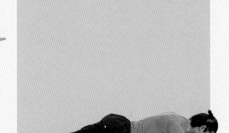

ⓟ CENTRE PLANK

p.58
Hold for 10 cycles of slow breathing

7

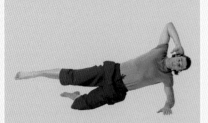

ⓟ THE SIDE KICK, KNEELING

p.66 (do on right side)
Do for 12–15 repetitions

8

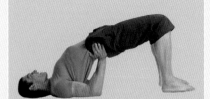

ⓟ ⓨ SHOULDER BRIDGE

p.63
Hold for 10 cycles of slow breathing

9

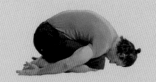

ⓨ CHILD'S POSE

p.81
Hold for as long as comfortable

10

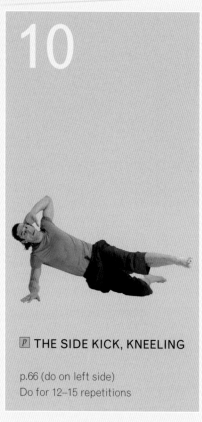

p THE SIDE KICK, KNEELING

p.66 (do on left side)
Do for 12–15 repetitions

11

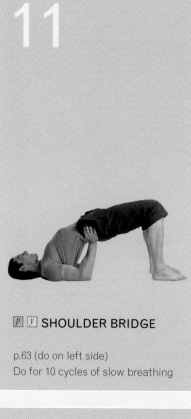

p y SHOULDER BRIDGE

p.63 (do on left side)
Do for 10 cycles of slow breathing

12

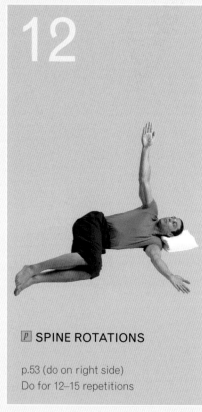

p SPINE ROTATIONS

p.53 (do on right side)
Do for 12–15 repetitions

16

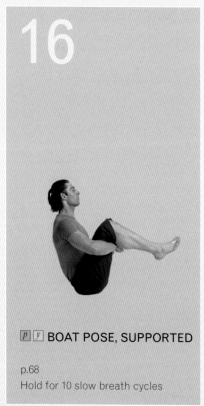

p y BOAT POSE, SUPPORTED

p.68
Hold for 10 slow breath cycles

17

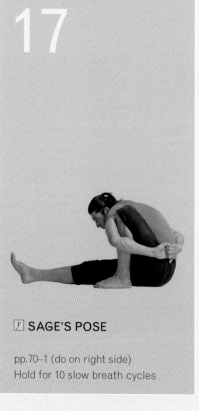

y SAGE'S POSE

pp.70–1 (do on right side)
Hold for 10 slow breath cycles

18

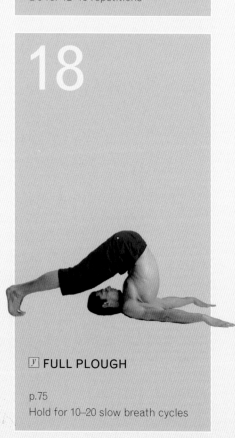

y FULL PLOUGH

p.75
Hold for 10–20 slow breath cycles

13

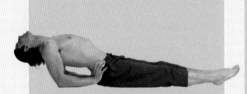

ⓨ SEATED HALF FISH

p.80
Hold for 5–10 slow breath cycles

14

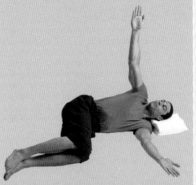

ⓟ SPINE ROTATIONS

p.53 (left side)
Do for 12–15 repetitions

15

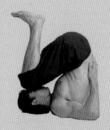

ⓨ HALF FOETUS, SUPPORTED

p.74
Hold for 10–20 slow breath cycles

19

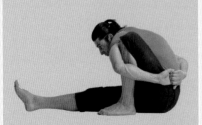

ⓨ SAGE'S POSE

pp.70–1 (left side)
Hold for 10 slow breath cycles

20

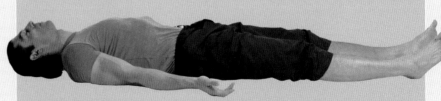

ⓨ RELAXATION

p.81
Rest for as long as necessary

30-minute "relaxed day" session

This 30-minute session contains different movements from the 15-minute version. It achieves the best results when practised at least twice a week alongside three 15-minute workouts. As it takes longer to complete, it is best to practise when you are relaxed and have more time. You can extend your workout time by staying in the Relaxation pose for longer or by doing more sets of your favourite exercises. Try to keep it flexible and just do what you can! This 30-minute session uses movements from the yoga vinyasa (see p.40), so read the breath instructions carefully and note that some steps are just transitions, and others are meant to be held.

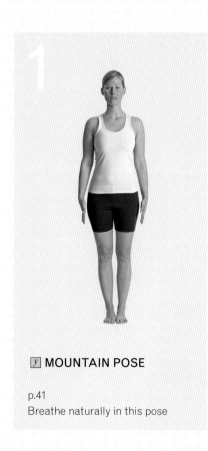

1

y MOUNTAIN POSE

p.41
Breathe naturally in this pose

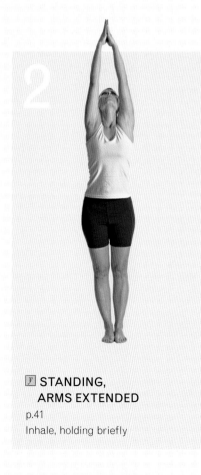

2

y STANDING,
   ARMS EXTENDED

p.41
Inhale, holding briefly

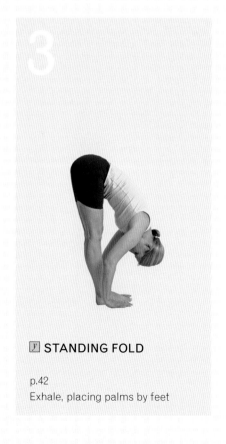

3

y STANDING FOLD

p.42
Exhale, placing palms by feet

4

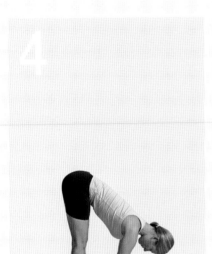

ⓨ ACTIVE BACK EXTENSION

p.42
Inhale, lengthening spine

5

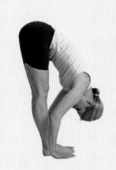

ⓨ STANDING FOLD

p.42
Exhale, placing palms by feet

6

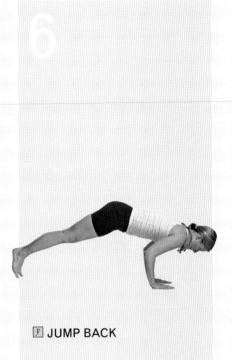

ⓨ JUMP BACK

p.43
Exhale, jumping legs back

7

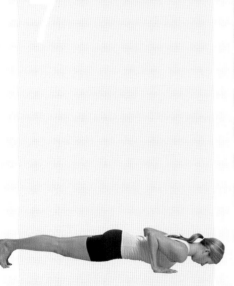

ⓨ ALL FOURS STAFF POSE

p.44
Same exhale as jump, bending arms

8

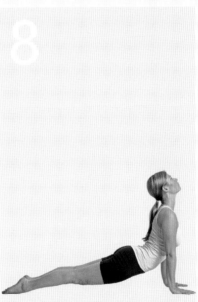

ⓨ UPWARD FACING DOG

p.45
Inhale, pushing chest forward

9

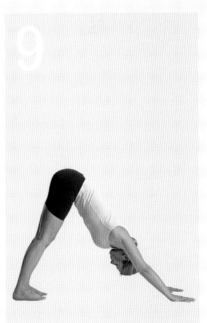

ⓨ DOWNWARD FACING DOG

p.46
Exhale, pushing up buttocks

10

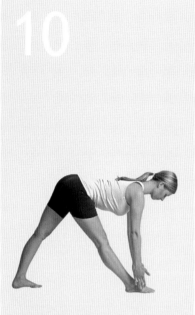

y **CLOSED PLANE
EXTENSION**

p.61
Hold for 5–10 slow breath cycles

11

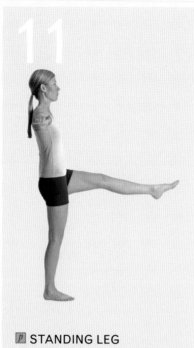

p **STANDING LEG
EXTENSION**

p.56 (on left side)
Do for 10–15 repetitions

12

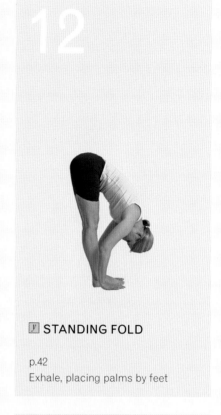

y **STANDING FOLD**

p.42
Exhale, placing palms by feet

16

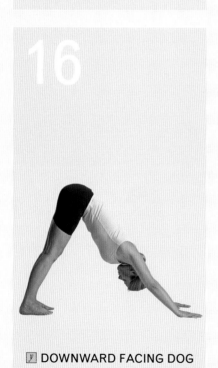

y **DOWNWARD FACING DOG**

p.46
Exhale, pushing up buttocks

17

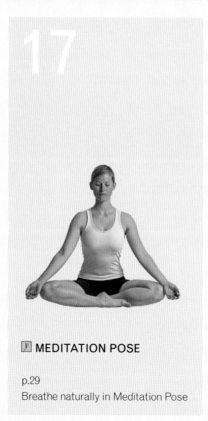

y **MEDITATION POSE**

p.29
Breathe naturally in Meditation Pose

18

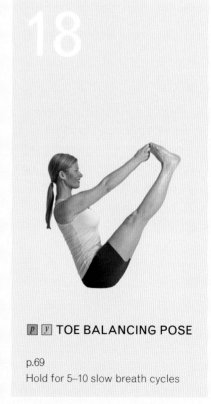

p *y* **TOE BALANCING POSE**

p.69
Hold for 5–10 slow breath cycles

13

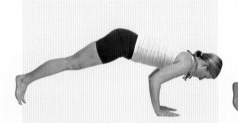

ⓨ JUMP BACK

p.43
Exhale, jumping legs back

14

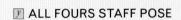

ⓨ ALL FOURS STAFF POSE

p.44
Same exhale as jump, bending arms

15

ⓨ UPWARD FACING DOG

p.45
Inhale, pushing chest forward

19

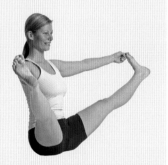

ⓟ ⓨ TOE BALANCING POSE

p.69 (harder alternative)
Hold for 5–10 slow breath cycles

20

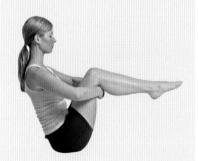

ⓟ THE ROLL

p.72
Do for 12–15 rolls

21

ⓟ THE SPINE STRETCH

p.67
Hold for 10 slow breath cycles

22

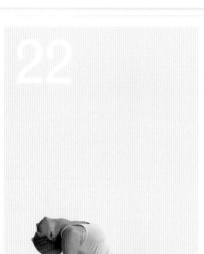

y SEATED HALF FISH

p.80 (easier alternative)
Do for 4–8 slow breath cycles

23

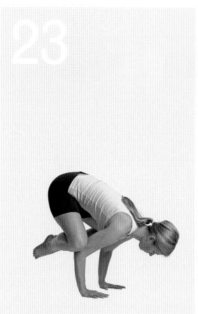

y BIRDIE

p.64
Hold for 4–10 slow breath cycles

24

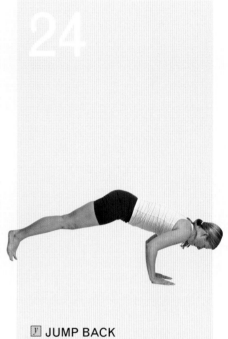

y JUMP BACK

p.43
Exhale, jumping legs back

28

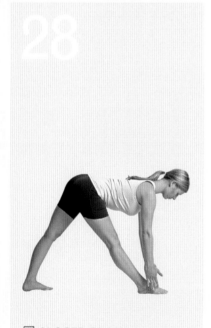

y CLOSED PLANE
EXTENSION

p.61
Hold for 5–10 slow breaths

29

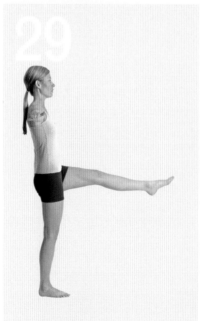

p STANDING LEG
EXTENSION

p.56 (on left side)
Do for 10–15 repetitions

30

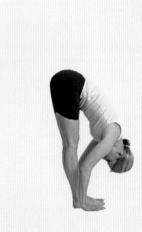

y STANDING FOLD

p.42
Exhale, placing palms by feet

25

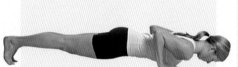

𝐲 ALL FOURS STAFF POSE

p.44
Same exhale as jump, bending arms

26

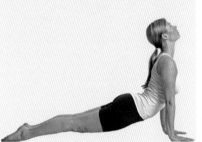

𝐲 UPWARD FACING DOG

p.45
Inhale, pushing chest forward

27

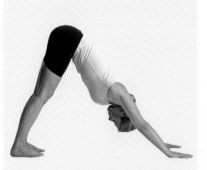

𝐲 DOWNWARD FACING DOG

p.46
Exhale, pushing up buttocks

31

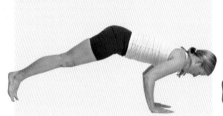

𝐲 JUMP BACK

p.43
Exhale, jumping legs back

32

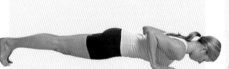

𝐲 ALL FOURS STAFF POSE

p.44
Same exhale as jump, bending arms

33

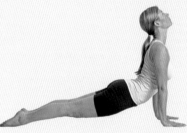

𝐲 UPWARD FACING DOG

p.45
Inhale, pushing chest forward

34

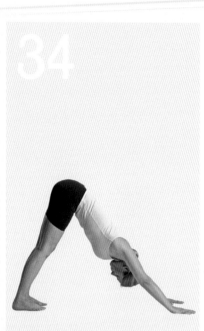

𝒚 DOWNWARD FACING DOG

p.46
Exhale, pushing up buttocks

35

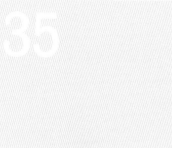
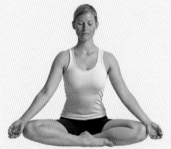

𝒚 MEDITATION POSE

p.29
Breathe naturally in meditation pose

36

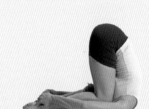

𝒚 FOETUS POSE

p.75
Hold for 10–15 slow breath cycles

37

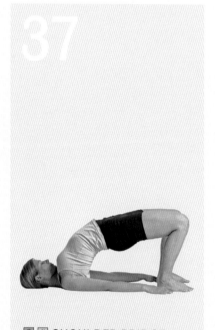

𝒑 𝒚 SHOULDER BRIDGE

p.63
Inhale, exhale and hold

38

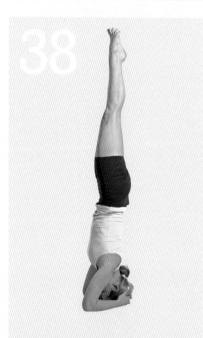

𝒚 HEADSTAND

pp.78–9
Practise slowly at your right level

39

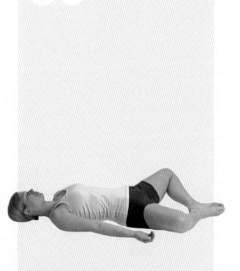

𝒑 𝒚 BUTTERFLY POSE

p.81
Breathe naturally

40

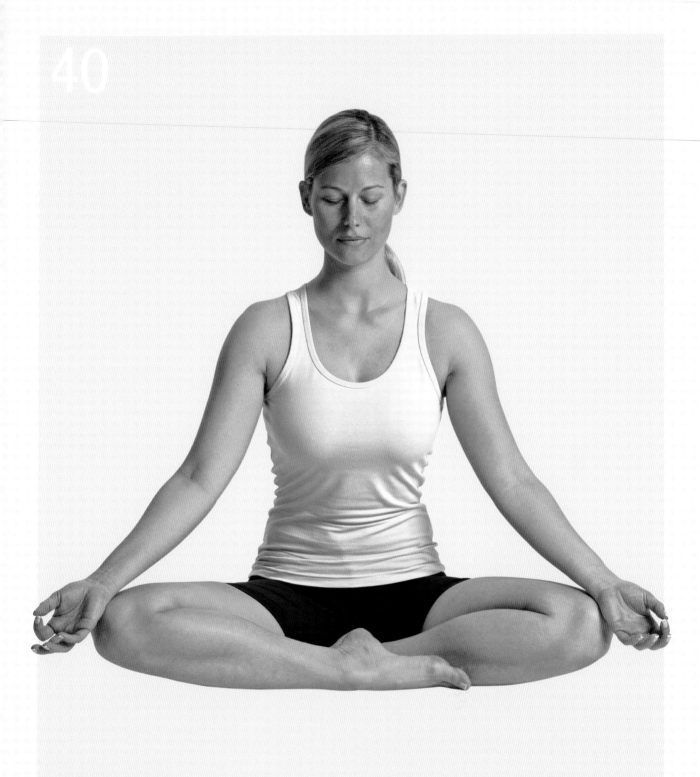

𝚢 MEDITATION POSE

p.29
Breathe naturally in Meditation Pose

Useful
Contacts

ASHTANGA YOGA RESEARCH INSTITUTE
Sri K. Pattabhi Jois
#235 8th Cross, 3rd Stage
Gokulam, Mysore 570002, Karnataka
India
Tel: +91 821 2516 756
www.ayri.org
Excellent centre where the author trained.

BAREFOOT STUDIO
Godfrey Devereux
3515 Old Cantrell Road
Little Rock, AR 72202
USA
Tel: +1 501 661 8005
www.barefootstudio.com
www.dynamicyogamerica.com
Workshops and retreats teaching Dynamic yoga.

BKS IYENGAR
Ramamani Iyengar Memorial Yoga
Institute (RIMYI)
1107 B/1 Hare Krishna Mandir Road,
Shivaji Nagar, Pune 411015,
Maharashtra.
India
Tel: +91 20 2565 6134
www.bksiyengar.com
A great teacher of Iyengar yoga.

THE DYNAMIC YOGA SCHOOL, ESSEX
Studio Suite, Roding Lane
Chigwell, Essex
UK
Tel: +44 (0) 7956 854 922
www.dynamicyogapilatesuk.com
The author's own yoga school which runs group and private courses, workshops, and retreats.

GILLIAN GREENWOOD
Body Control Pilates Training
Organisation
Tel: +44 (0) 20 7385 3577
www.gilliangreenwood.com
Private, group, pre-natal and post-natal pilates classes in West London.

THE PILATES INSTITUTE LONDON (MICHAEL KING)
Wimborne House
151–155 New North Road
London N1 6TA
UK
Tel: +44 (0)20 7253 3177
www.pilates-institute.com
No longer running courses, but this is an informative website.

PILATES METHOD ALLIANCE
PO Box 370906
Miami, FL 33137-0906
USA
Tel: +1 866 573 4945
www.pilatesmethodalliance.org
Information on locating pilates schools and associations in the USA and worldwide.

SANTA MONICA YOGA
1640 Ocean Park Blvd.
Santa Monica, CA 90405
USA
Tel: +1 310 396 4040
www.santamonicayoga.com
Classes and workshops.

JOHN SCOTT YOGA
The Yoga Studio
The Old Newlyn School, 3–4
off Kenstella Road
Newlyn
Penzance TR18 5AB
UK
www.johnscottashtanga.co.uk
Great teacher offering international retreats and Cornwall-based workshops.

UNITED STATES YOGA ASSOCIATION
2159 Filbert Street
San Francisco, CA 94123
USA
Tel: +1 415 931 YOGA
www.usyoga.org
Athletic or hatha yoga teaching.

WINDFIRE YOGA RETREATS
Godfrey Devereux
Villa Casalecchi
Umbria
Italy
www.windfireyoga.com
The author's teacher, offering great Dynamic yoga retreats worldwide.

Author acknowledgments

This book was a journey travelled by many special people through some of the most beautiful places. To my husband, Anthony, whose giant shoulders I stand upon – I salute you. I am deeply grateful to Godfrey Devereux for sharing his rugged honesty and for empowering his own practice – the significance of your contribution shines back to you in the thousands of students that you reach.

To the beautiful Maria José Santelices, my spiritual sister, for loving life and inspiring those around you. Wiggle Wiggle. To Lili, for never accepting the impossible. The sun will always shine for you.

To Virginie, for sharing her beautiful yoga practice, to Sally, for a smile to light the darkest of days, and to Jon, for standing by his word. To Yolande Green and all those at Mitchell Beazley who helped to bring this book into the real hands of real people. To Jill, my mother, who makes it clear to me that the completion of this book is not the end of anything, it's just the beginning. To Claire Bloom and Stuart Best for supporting my vision.

A thousand salutations to every single person that has attended my classes, workshops, or retreats or have purchased a video or book. Those who have shared with me the powerful testimony of the value that my work has had in their lives gives us all a reason to continue on our journey. Your support of my work means more to me than I could ever possibly put into words. I dedicate this book to you.